About the Author

Susan Saunders is a TV producer, writer and health coach. Through one-to-one coaching, workshops and classes, she helps people across the world age well. She's also co-author of best-seller, *The Age-Well Project*.

Find the latest research on ageing well at
agewellproject.com
and details of coaching, online courses and events at
susansaundershealth.com

THE
AGE
WELL
PLAN

The 6-Week Programme to Kickstart
a Longer, Healthier, Happier Life

Susan Saunders

The co-author of *The Age-Well Project*

PIATKUS

PIATKUS

First published in Great Britain in 2020 by Piatkus

1 3 5 7 9 10 8 6 4 2

A CIP catalogue record for this book
is available from the British Library.

ISBN 978-0-349-42553-5

Typeset in Sabon by M Rules
Printed and bound in Great Britain by Clays Ltd, Elcograf, S.p.A.

Papers used by Piatkus are from well-managed forests
and other responsible sources.

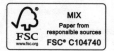

Piatkus
An imprint of
Little, Brown Book Group
Carmelite House
50 Victoria Embankment
London EC4Y 0DZ

An Hachette UK Company
www.hachette.co.uk

www.littlebrown.co.uk

To Richard, for showing me that love and laughter
really are the best medicine.

Contents

Acknowledgements

I stand on the shoulders of giants – the doctors and researchers who dedicate their lives to understanding how and why we age, and what we can do about it. Everyone who's ever sat at a bench in a lab, stared into microscope or written a paper that has deepened our understanding of the ageing process has helped make this book possible.

I owe a debt of gratitude to the experts I interviewed for this book, Dr Stephan Rechtschaffen, Dr Lori Shemek, Myra Robson, Jane Baker, Dr Scott Cairney, Marta Zaraska and Professor Carol Brayne. Thank you for sharing your knowledge and time with me.

Huge thanks to my fabulous and inspiring Age-Well Project partner-in-crime, Annabel Streets, for encouraging this next step along the path, and our agent Rachel Mills, who said 'Yes!' when this book was a mere paragraph, and who nurtured it into being. Thanks also to the team at Rachel Mills Literary for their seamless work behind the scenes.

I'm extremely grateful to the editorial team at Piatkus: Jillian Stewart, Jan Cutler and, most especially, Zoe Bohm for her infectious enthusiasm and guiding hand on the tiller. Thanks also to the wider team and to Beth Wright for spreading the word on all things Age Well.

My family, Richard, Honor and Unity, can't be thanked

enough for putting up with me yelling 'I've got a *book* to write' every time they needed something, for eating almost all the vegetables I put in front of them, and for surrounding me with love, laughter and encouragement.

Gratitude to the many friends who have cheered me along the way. From supporting me through the dark days of my mother's dementia diagnosis right through to helping me choose the cover for this book, thank you for being with me.

Most importantly, this book is inspired by the followers of the Age-Well Project on the blog and social media; all those who left a comment, asked a question, came to a masterclass, attended a workshop, joined my coaching programme, and everyone else I've met along the way who wants to age well. I salute you.

INTRODUCTION

Who am I, and why am I here?

For the best part of a decade I've been on a mission to age well, learning how to reduce my risk of the chronic conditions of ageing. I wasn't always interested in my health – drinking, smoking (eek!) and rarely exercising in my hedonistic twenties. In my thirties and early forties, I found myself sandwiched between very young children and a mother with dementia, so my own wellbeing slipped way down the list. But I've turned my health around since then and now I want to share what I've learnt with you.

For the next six weeks I'm here to guide you towards your own age-well future. I'm excited that we're going to create your age-well plan together, so that you can take control of your health now and in the years to come.

Together we'll transform your health and mindset. In six weeks' time you'll have created your own age-well plan, which will carry you into the future with abundant good health. Every simple, powerful action that I suggest in this book I do myself, and each one is backed by science. Ageing well isn't some weirdo wellness fad with green juice and extreme diets. It's tiny tweaks to your daily routine that add up to radically reclaiming your health.

By creating your own age-well plan, you're going to achieve:

- A reduced risk of the chronic diseases of ageing.
- Bespoke health goals that work for you.
- Powerful age-well strategies that fit into *every* day – without them taking *all* day.
- An understanding of the science of longevity and cellular ageing.
- Improved immunity to illness.
- Increased energy levels and better fitness.
- More regular, restful sleep.
- A mindset to help you face the future with positivity.
- An environment in which you can age well.

As a health coach, and one half of the Age-Well Project, I teach clients and workshop groups how to make the most of the years ahead. Time and time again I've seen people have the a-ha! moment when they think: *I can do that* or *I can fit that into my life.* I'd like you to have those moments, too, when you realise that you can achieve the changes needed to age well.

One workshop attendee told me that learning to age well had changed her life. I want that for you as well.

My story

My age-well plan began with a family tragedy.

I was 36 years old with a toddler, a newborn, a husband and a house to take care of, as well as a full-time job. I felt pretty stretched, and life was a constant juggle. Then my mother was diagnosed with severe dementia. My world was turned upside down: not only was I a mum, a wife and a colleague, but now I was a carer too. I'm an only child, and my dad died a long time ago, so there was no one else to turn to. What made this even harder to bear was that, as a teenager, I'd watched my mum going through the same thing with her own mother.

I cared for my mum for 12 years. That toddler and newborn were teenagers by the time she died and I realised I'd do anything to reduce the chances of my daughters having to look after me in the future. I began studying scientific research on healthy ageing, and overhauling my diet, exercise regime, sleep, engagement with the world and the environment around me.

This research led to the blog I write with my friend, Annabel Streets, at agewellproject.com. Annabel has a similar story to mine and the same fascination with the science of ageing well. The blog grew into a best-selling book on longevity, *The Age-Well Project*.

Discovering how to age well has transformed my life so completely that I realised I had to help others gain the same benefits. I qualified as a health coach and now help people all over the world enjoy the years to come feeling fit and fabulous. The six-week plan contained in this book grew out of the realisation that my coaching experience could help you to make ageing well a daily reality, transforming your life.

How to use this book

You might be reading this book because you want to make the most of everything the future has to offer, but you're confused by all the conflicting advice out there. Or perhaps you have read *The Age-Well Project* and learnt a lot from it, but you're wondering how to make it work in your own life. You know your life could be healthier, but you lack motivation. I know how you feel – I've been there. With that in mind, I've designed this plan to take you step by step through ageing well. Every action that I suggest to you, I do myself. And I've done the research to know why it works.

This book will help you to prioritise the strategies you need and find the motivation to build them into your daily life. You'll create a specific, individualised plan at your pace, and on your budget, to help you build healthy habits for the rest of your life. There's lots of space for you to journal your own thoughts and ideas, and to monitor your progress. (But if you prefer not to write in the book, buy a small notebook to use instead.) In six weeks' time you will have laid out a plan for the years to come – and you'll feel amazing right now!

Each week you'll get to grips with a different element of ageing well to build on the previous weeks of the plan. By Week 6 you will have created a new age-well lifestyle that's easy to continue forever:

Week 1 How to plan: understand the science of getting older, create your purpose in ageing well and get to know your ageing body.

Week 2 How to eat: junk processed foods, get back into the kitchen and feel the power of plants (plus, chocolate!).

Week 3 How to move: work movement into every hour of every day, exercise the most important muscle of all and have fun while you're doing it.

Week 4 How to sleep: create a positive sleep environment, get into a bedtime routine and make blue light work for you.

Week 5 How to 'be': feel positive about getting older, appreciate the joy of novelty and understand why friends come with age-well benefits.

Week 6 How to live: make an age-well home, deal with environmental toxins and think about your future.

Week 1 has a slightly different format from the rest of the book in order to lay firm foundations for the coming weeks. It's all about creating your personal plan and the mindset to achieve your goals. After that, each week follows the same format:

The big picture You will find five essential lessons to help you prioritise changes in your own life, plus the scientific research that explains each one. It is much easier to stick to a health goal when you understand the scientific basis for it. And I've laid out what I do: the tricks and tips that work best for me.

The Top 10 are the non-negotiable daily actions to work into your life. Ten might sound like a lot, but some take absolutely no time (stand on one leg while you clean your teeth, for example), and some fulfil multiple roles – a morning walk ticks off to-dos from three sections of the book!

Your age-well week Not every action needs to be implemented every day. Work these straightforward tips into your week for extra age-well benefits. The week is super-flexible – and always remember it's *your* age-well plan.

How to make it work This includes the resources you need – from larder lists to sleep trackers.

Your personal age-well plan This is where you build your own plan. There are questionnaires and checklists to fill out, plus space to journal and set your intentions for ageing well (or you can use a notebook instead). Writing down our intentions makes us far more likely to stick to them. Each week I'll ask you to spell out how you're going to age well from now on. This is your commitment to yourself to make your future as fabulous as possible.

You can take the plan step by step or dip into the areas where you feel you need the most support. But, crucially, just start: you're building a plan that will last you for the rest of your life.

The importance of habits and mindset

Simple daily habits, ingrained in our lives, can make all the difference to how well we age. They have a cumulative effect, each reinforcing the other. Creating a routine around positive activities is itself beneficial.

Ageing well takes focus and small changes each day. There's no quick fix. I can't promise that in six weeks' time you'll have lost 3.2kg (7lb) or 5cm (2in) off your waist (although you might – but that's not why we're here). I can't promise you that six weeks from now you'll have dodged the bullet on cancer, Alzheimer's or diabetes. But you'll have reduced your risk of all those conditions, and you'll have started to build a lifetime of healthy habits. Many of the illnesses and impediments that we associate with old age take root in midlife, only revealing themselves decades later. It's never too late to begin, and you're not a lost cause, but the time to start making changes is *now*.

Your mindset – the behaviours that affect the way we take action – will make all the difference as you begin your plan.

Do an audit of how you feel about ageing: what do you believe is possible? Does your mindset support your goal of ageing well? Tune into the idea of creating your age-well plan and how it's going to help you achieve healthy longevity.

Throughout this book there are opportunities for you to decide which actions are best for you, and to incorporate them into your own daily life. As I've learnt more about the science of longevity, I've overhauled my mindset and my own routines to make my life an age-well one. These are straightforward changes that take little time: I still go to work every day and take care of my family. You can do the same. In six weeks' time you'll have a blueprint for an age-well life that works for you.

How I start and end my age-well day, every day

Morning:

- A six-minute workout
- A hot–cold–hot shower (find out why I hum in the shower on page 188)
- Black coffee or tea
- A few moments of gratitude, meditation or mindfulness
- Breaking my fast mid-morning – not first thing
- Thirty minutes of daylight (see page 119 for why that's important)

Evening:

- A digital detox
- Dim the lights after 9pm
- Brush my teeth standing on alternate legs
- Read a book
- Pink noise (discover what this is on page 151)

Why you can make a difference – and why you should

The evidence that a healthy lifestyle improves our chances of ageing well is overwhelming. Thousands of scientific reports have decoded how living well leads to an increased healthspan (the years of good health we have, as opposed to living with illness or a chronic condition). Here's just one example: research published in January 2020 in the *British Medical Journal*[1] credited 'low-risk lifestyle factors' (not smoking, not being overweight, getting 30 minutes of moderate to vigorous exercise a day, a moderate alcohol intake, a good-quality, Mediterranean-style diet) with an extra ten years of healthspan. Sounds good, doesn't it?

It was the possibility of increasing our healthspan that fascinated Annabel and me when we started the Age-Well Project. We've been overwhelmed by the response to the first book, by the community that's grown up around our blog and by the number of people who want to age well. This Age-Well Plan grew out of the realisation that I could offer more guidance on how to make the Age-Well Project work, day by day, week by week.

Putting healthy behaviours into practice can be tough, which is why we're going to work on it together for the next six weeks. There are no guarantees, of course. In the years to come, some of us will be felled by diseases and conditions over which we have little control; others will become spritely centenarians. If the coronavirus pandemic has taught us anything, it's that being in good health gives us resilience to disease, adversity and unexpected change. We should all give ourselves the best opportunity to age well, whatever our starting point.

Most importantly, by starting to age well now, you'll start to feel great now, too. All the practices, ideas and tips in this book will have an immediate effect on your health. When we started the Age-Well Project I was so focused on my future health that the here-and-now benefits rather took me by surprise. I'm very glad they did!

As you create your own age-well plan, remember that you're not alone. The age-well community is here to cheer you on. If you want to let us know how your plan is going, turn to page 236 for our social network pages and join us.

Let's get started.

A health warning

I'm not a doctor, scientist or dietician. I'm here to guide you to make your own healthy choices, based on my research, and coach you to discover what's best for you.

My suggestions are not a substitute for medical advice from a doctor. If you have an illness or chronic condition, a health professional should be your first port of call.

A note on research

Many thousands of studies have delved into the ageing process and what might extend our healthspan. I've tried to focus on the latest research, particularly that published since we wrote *The Age-Well Project*: large longitudinal studies, tracking the health of extensive cohorts over a long time, and independently funded research.

These reports often reach a conclusion about a 'risk factor' – the possibility that a particular action might increase or decrease our risk of a specific illness or condition. Sometimes the results are dramatic, with risk factors increasing or decreasing by a large percentage. But bear in mind that your initial risk might be very low. If your risk for a particular cancer is just 5 per cent, increasing it by 20 per cent only takes your overall risk to 6 per cent.

WEEK 1

How to Plan

Week 1 is all about creating the mindset to age well – starting today and continuing for the rest of your life. This is where you start to take responsibility for how you age. It doesn't matter what the starting point is, it's beginning the journey that's important. You might be struggling with a range of health conditions, or you may be super-fit and want to feel even better. There's an age-well plan for everyone.

The 'why, what, who?' of ageing

You'll spend this week learning how we age and evaluating your current health and future risk factors. You'll get clear on your intentions: why you want to age well and where you need to focus, creating your own personalised age-well plan as you go.

I call it the 'why, what, who?' of ageing:

Why? Why are you here? What's brought you to this book? You want to age well, but who and/or what are you doing it for? Having a sense of purpose as we age has been found to reduce mortality risk. The long-lived Japanese call it *ikigai*, literally 'reason for being'. You're going to find yours.

What? What's ageing you from the outside? And what's happening inside your body as you get older? I'm going to give you a basic understanding of the science of ageing: what's happening at a cellular level as the years go by. You'll find it much easier to stick to lifestyle changes once you understand how they benefit your ageing body, I promise!

Who? Who are you as you age? What have you inherited in your genetic make-up, and what are your personal risk factors? We're going to interrogate those issues so that you can decide exactly where you need to focus as you personalise your plan.

Understanding my own sense of purpose, the science of ageing and my key risk factors keeps me motivated with my age-well plan. Now it's time to work on yours.

Assess yourself as you start the week

Don't worry if you don't know the answers to the questions below; this week is all about finding them. I want you to be able to track your progress and to pat yourself on the back in a week's time!

Questionnaire: knowing your body as you age

		Yes	No
1	Do you have a clear sense of why you want to age well?	☐	☐
2	Do you understand the external processes ageing you?	☐	☐
3	Do you understand how you are ageing at a cellular level?	☐	☐
4	Do you know what your forebears died of, and any illnesses that they might have had before they died?	☐	☐
5	Do you know your:		
	BMI?	☐	☐
	Waist-to-hip measurement?	☐	☐
	Blood pressure?	☐	☐
	Resting heart rate?	☐	☐
	Cholesterol level?	☐	☐
	Blood glucose levels?	☐	☐

Your score:

If you have lots of 'no's, and don't know all the information about your health, it's not a problem. I'll be explaining how to find it and why it is important, throughout this chapter.

By the end of this week you will:

- Be motivated to age well with a clear sense of purpose.
- Have set your intention for ageing well.

- Understand the exterior factors that contribute to ageing.
- Know what's happening in your body at a cellular level as you age.
- Reveal possible patterns and issues in your genetic history.
- Evaluate your own key markers of ageing.
- Focus on priorities for your age-well plan.

The big picture: why are you here? Your purpose as you age

Your mind is the most important age-well tool that you have: it gives you the power to plan for the future you want and the strength to go after it. Scientific research backs this: a 2019 study of almost 7,000 people found that those with the strongest sense of purpose had decreased mortality rates.[1] Heart, circulatory and blood conditions were noticeably reduced among those who lived purposefully. The researchers defined 'purpose' as 'a self-organising life aim that stimulates goals, promotes healthy behaviours and gives meaning to life'.

I need you to consider *why* you want to age well. Over the next six weeks you're going to make major shifts in how you eat, move, sleep, think and live. To stay motivated, you need to set an intention that inspires you to make these changes. This is purpose: it drives us to create a satisfying future, and it helps us to get the most from the things we achieve – large and small – right now. It will help us set our priorities in the coming weeks.

On page 16 there's space for you to write down your purpose: the reason you are striving to age well. Think about what will nurture your unique skills and talents and make you truly *you*. Perhaps you want to climb a mountain, move to Australia, nurture a garden, be the best grandparent ever. Perhaps you want to help others, improve your community or inspire change. Perhaps you want to be the world's oldest pole dancer. It really doesn't matter what that intention is, and it's not necessarily something you'll go and find, or an activity you 'should' be doing, it's what will make you feel whole. Most importantly, your sense of purpose is whatever will inspire you to stick to your own age-well plan.

Like most of us, I know I need to take care of my health if I want to age well. But what really keeps me eating the green veg and turning up at the gym is knowing that, cumulatively, these actions increase the chances that I will be able to live out my purpose.

This is the purpose that keeps me on track with my age-well plan:

> 'To help the world age well; to remain healthy myself
> so that I can travel, enjoying arts and culture around
> the world, for as long as I can.'

Here are a couple of examples from the experts in this book to help you on your way:

> 'My purpose is to promote the benefits of healthy, strong
> feet throughout life so people can participate in a full life.
> I'll lead by example, keeping my feet and body healthy for
> as long as possible to get out in nature.'
>
> **Jane Baker, Harley Street foot and ankle**
> **specialist physio, see page 123**

'My purpose is to do my modest share in preventing cat-
astrophic climate change so that my child, and all other
young people, can still enjoy our beautiful planet in the
future in a relatively unchanged state.'

**Marta Zaraska, science writer
and author, see page 195**

Now it's your turn. What's your purpose? What's going to keep
you motivated and able to stick to your age-well plan. Write
it out here:

Where else can you write your purpose so that you will remember it? Write it out again and stick it onto the fridge or tuck it
into your wallet. Put it anywhere you'll see it regularly. Read
it out to your family or share it on social media – and tag the
Age-Well Project if you do! Sharing our purpose motivates us
to stay on track.

What's ageing you?

How you age is dictated by a combination of internal and
external factors. This is not about blame: you can't control
all these factors, but you can control some of them, or at least
mitigate them. Understanding what they are, and their impact
on your health as you age, is key to staying on track with your
age-well plan.

10 toxic risk factors for ageing from the outside in

1 **Smoking** Hold it right there – if you smoke, please put down this book and seek the help you need to quit. Then come back and let's carry on. Smoking increases your risk of developing more than 50 serious health conditions,[2] and increases the risk of dying from all causes by up to two-thirds.[3]

2 **Bad diet** They say that you can't outrun a bad diet. However healthy the rest of your lifestyle, what you eat trumps everything. A poor diet impacts all the chronic conditions of ageing, and it directly contributes to an increased risk of diabetes and obesity.

3 **Excess weight** More than one-third of adults in England are overweight and a further 29 per cent are obese. Obesity accelerates the rate at which we get old by impacting all the key hallmarks of the ageing process (see page 56).[4]

4 **Sedentary behaviour** We spend between nine and 12 hours a day sitting down, and it's killing us. The World Health Organization (WHO) ranks sedentary behaviour among the 10 leading causes of death. Lack of movement day to day is linked to an increased risk of some cancers and cognitive decline as well as weight gain and overall morbidity.

5 **Stress** When I was caring for my mum, raising small children and working full time, I was stressed *all*

the time. A study by the Mental Health Foundation found that three-quarters of those questioned had felt so stressed in the previous year that they were over-whelmed or unable to cope.[5] Stress is a risk factor for many of the conditions of ageing, such as heart disease, dementia, diabetes and cancer.

6   **Lack of sleep** Just when we need sleep most, in midlife and beyond, it eludes us. Over the age of 50, our circa-dian rhythms (the internal 24-hour clock that governs waking and sleeping) change, making it harder to fall asleep and easier to wake up at night. And that's on top of the wakefulness engendered by modern life: bright lights from our screens, Netflix binge watching, a flood of emails to answer. Chronic sleep loss increases the risk of heart disease, diabetes and cognitive decline.

7   **Over-consumption of alcohol** This isn't one of those health books which tells you to stop drinking altogether. Numerous studies have shown that a moderate amount of alcohol can be beneficial as we age. But more than 14 units a week is classed as heavy drinking, and is linked to higher dementia risk, decreased immune response, bone loss and increased mortality.

8   **Air pollution** Ninety per cent of the world's population breathes unacceptably high levels of pollution, accord-ing to the WHO. Dirty air has been linked in recent years to accelerated rates of Alzheimer's, cardiovascular disease and depression.[6] It's estimated that polluted air reduces the life expectancy of Europeans by two years.[7]

9 **Toxins and plastics** The food and drink we ingest
   are doused in toxic chemicals from pesticides, plastics, solvents and cleaning agents. Many of these can
   damage our DNA, ageing us at the most basic cellular
   level. The average person might ingest 100,000 pieces
   of microplastics, weighing around 250g, each year.[8]
   Research into the impact of microplastics on ageing is
   in its infancy but, unsurprisingly, results indicate that
   ingesting plastics isn't doing us any good.

10 **Loneliness** The number of over-fifties experiencing
   loneliness in the UK is set to reach two million by 2025,
   a 49 per cent increase in 10 years. Being alone doesn't
   just feel miserable; it impacts health, too. Loneliness
   increases the risk of death by 29 per cent, with lonely
   people more likely to suffer from dementia, heart disease and depression.

Take some time this week to identify which of these factors most
impact your life. There's space at the end of this chapter to write
them down. Please don't over-stress if you are impacted by many
of the factors listed above: we'll tackle them in the coming weeks.

A word about menopause

Everyone woman who lives long enough will experience the
menopause. The symptoms can be debilitating, and can last
for many years. If you're experiencing menopause symptoms
that are hard to manage, get help from your GP in the first

instance. No woman should ever suffer in silence. This isn't a book about menopause – there are plenty of terrific tomes out there which cover the subject. The most important thing, from an age-well perspective, is to have a well-managed menopause (however you choose to do that) so that you can focus on healthy longevity going forward.

Understanding cellular ageing

This is the science bit, so buckle up. Understanding what's happening in your body as you age is a critical part of your Week 1 planning and preparation. Only then can you appreciate the relevance of the choices you make around what you eat, how you move, sleep and live. Co-creating the Age-Well Project, and training as a health coach, meant that I had to take a deep dive into the science of ageing. But I've found the knowledge empowering; it keeps me motivated to stay on track with a healthy lifestyle.

Ageing happens at a cellular level. We're familiar with the exterior signs of ageing: the grey hair, wrinkles and sagginess gifted to us by the years. Inside each cell of our bodies, a similar process is underway: DNA damage, mitochondrial decline, telomere shortening, inflammation and oxidative stress all take their toll. (I'll explain all these terms and why we want to reduce their impact on our bodies.)

There's no one scientific theory that explains the entire process of ageing, and research is still incomplete in many areas. But scientists now believe that how we age comes down to a combination of factors, known as the nine hallmarks of ageing, which occur as a result of biologically programmed decline and cumulative damage within our cells.[9] There is a genetic component, but these interconnected hallmarks are all impacted by environmental factors and lifestyle: we *can* change the way we age at a cellular level.

I've tried to simplify the key issues but it's a lot to take on board, so do read this section more than once if you need to.

9 toxic risk factors for ageing from the inside out

1   **DNA instability** DNA is found in the nucleus of every cell and it's what makes us us. DNA molecules are the hereditary material in our genes; we get half from each parent. Throughout our lives, DNA continuously replicates and divides to create new cells when our bodies need them. As we get older, interior and exterior factors challenge our DNA, resulting in errors in the original genetic code. Imagine copying the same book by hand, over and over again. In time, you'd be bound to make mistakes – that's what happens as our DNA replicates.

2   **Telomere shortening** Our DNA molecules are packaged into thread-like structures called chromosomes. Think of chromosomes like shoelaces. The tip on the end stops the shoelace from fraying: telomeres do the same job for our chromosomes. As DNA replicates, telomeres wear down, making it difficult for the shoelace-like chromosomes to function properly. Eventually they 'fray' like old shoelaces and die. Forget the number of candles on

your birthday cake, the clearest indication of your true age is the length of your telomeres. The shorter they are, the older you are.

3 **Epigenetic alterations** Our genome (the sum total of our DNA) comes with an instruction manual, the epigenome, which controls how genes are expressed. This expression of genes switches them on and off, allowing DNA to create a huge variety of cells in our bodies. The epigenome attaches chemical compounds and proteins to DNA, marking it so that it knows how to make heart cells or fingernail cells, for example, from the same raw material. The epigenome also has a huge range of repair mechanisms primed and ready to deal with DNA damage. But, over time, these can fail, exhausted by errors in the replication of our genetic code, as well as exterior factors such as lifestyle and pollution. This can lead to the epigenome making mistakes, switching the wrong genes on and off.

4 **Protein misfolding** Every one of our cells contains thousands of protein molecules, which perform a wide variety of functions within the cell. These proteins are neatly folded into shape so that they can do their work, but stresses inside and outside the body cause them to unfold. The body either refolds the proteins back into shape or, if they're too damaged, gobbles them up in a process called autophagy (literally, self-eating).[10] Ageing impairs the system that identifies and tags proteins for this recycling process, and without this quality control damaged proteins build up. This has been linked to

heart disease[11] and the accumulation of damaged proteins in the brain, which causes Alzheimer's disease.

5 **Nutritional insensitivity** Our cells can 'read' how much fat or glucose we have in our bodies and respond accordingly, burning or storing fat. As we age, that system becomes less sensitive, impacting the storage of fat, and the response of insulin to glucose. The end result is weight gain and, potentially, diabetes.

6 **Mitochondrial function** Every cell in our bodies runs on 'batteries' called mitochondria: structures which convert energy from food into a form that cells can use. This conversion process produces waste in the form of free radicals. These unpaired electrons are unstable, and wreak havoc in our bodies. When we're younger they're mopped up by antioxidants (molecules which generously donate electrons to free radicals) and the damage is minimal. As we age, they build up, causing oxidative stress. On a car, we'd call it rust. We're rusting! The build-up of this 'rust' in our cellular batteries makes them less efficient.

7 **Zombie cells** When our cells can no longer cope with all this DNA damage, stress and rusting they give up the ghost and become 'senescent': zombie cells that refuse to die and cause further harm by pumping out inflammation. Inflammation is both our body's best friend and its worst enemy. If we cut ourselves, the body sends an acute inflammatory response and our skin is red and swollen as the cut heals. But as we age, the body

is almost permanently in a threat state, dealing with ageing cells and broken DNA. This chronic, low-grade inflammation alters communication within each cell and is a hallmark of ageing – so much so that doctors have coined the term 'inflamm-ageing'. It's linked to type-2 diabetes, cognitive decline, reduced immunity, cancer and cardiovascular disease. High levels of inflammation are found in people who become frail in old age.

8 **Stem-cell exhaustion** Stem cells are brand-new cells with factory settings that our epigenome can program to replace any cell in the body if it becomes damaged. As we get older, they run out of energy and fail to renew or replace other damaged cells properly. This is part of the reason that injuries take longer to heal as we get older.

9 **Altered cell communication** Our cells are in constant communication with each other, passing messages back and forth so that they can function normally. As we age, messages become harder to decipher and cells fail to respond to messages they receive. With all this background noise, the immune system can no longer clear out damaged cells or respond appropriately to viruses, leaving us at greater risk of cancer or infections. Hormonal messaging – from insulin, for example – gets lost, too.

This sounds like an awful lot of things going wrong, doesn't it? But there are two key points to take from it:

1 Ageing is a natural process, hardwired into our genes. Some of us will age better than others, some of us will get ill, some of us won't.

2 We can alter the way our genes express themselves and improve these ageing hallmarks.

The good news

Although we inherit our genes from our parents, the way they behave within our bodies isn't carved in stone. The epigenome decides how genes are expressed, and that can be influenced by environmental and biological factors. We might be able to control the risk of an inherited predisposition, to a greater or lesser extent, by our lifestyle.

In recent years, there have been huge leaps forward in our understanding of what can switch on, and switch off, the cellular processes that result in ageing. Major findings include what scientists refer to as 'longevity pathways', which the epigenome uses to regulate DNA behaviour. These pathways are involved in an array of different processes, including metabolism, cognition and stress response.[12] They are signalling systems that send instructions to cells, telling them what to do next.

The hard work of switching genes on and off all the time is done by a family of enzymes called sirtuins. They work across multiple cellular pathways that regulate gene expression, ageing, immune function, DNA repair, telomere length and metabolism. Sirtuins are the paramedics of the epigenome, rushing to the scene to repair damaged DNA. Sirtuin activity declines with age, so the repair mechanisms falter, which is why we are more prone to illnesses and viruses as we get older.

We're able to boost sirtuin activity, however, by what we eat and what we do. Keeping the repair process functioning allows us to deal with the external and internal damage of growing older, creating the conditions we need to age well.

Throughout the book, as I talk about what we eat, how we move and what we do, I'll link back to these cellular processes so that you can understand how your actions directly impact the ageing process. Use this powerful knowledge as you create your own age-well plan.

A word about the immune system and ageing well

The coronavirus pandemic has thrown a harsh spotlight on the health of our older population. The relationship between our immune systems and our ageing bodies is a complex one: all the hallmarks of ageing listed above impact, and are impacted by, the immune system. Put simply, the production and function of vital immune cells decreases as we age, so we are not able to respond to immune challenges as robustly as we could when we were younger.[13] Throughout this book I've referenced actions which can help support our immune systems as we age.

Who are you as you age?

We've explored what's ageing you and why you want to age well, but do you know *how* you're ageing? We spend so much of our adult lives thinking about others – partners, children, parents, bosses and colleagues – that we rarely take the time to stop and think about ourselves. How well do you know the ageing you?

Your genetic history

It's easy to think that we'll age just like our forebears, with the thought process going something like this: *My mum/dad/aunt/ granddad had dementia/arthritis/diabetes/cancer, so I expect that I'll get it, too.* The reality is that much of how we age, and our risk of developing age-related illnesses, is related to lifestyle and environmental factors. This is tremendously empowering, as we saw on page 25. Genes are an important part of the story, however.

Roughly – very roughly – 20 to 30 per cent of how we age is down to the genes we've inherited from our ancestors. Scientists know this from studies of twins which show that a shared gene pool doesn't result in identical ageing patterns.

Understanding what we might, or might not, have inherited from our ancestors is important as we create our own age-well plans, to give us focus. Knowing that both my mum and grandmother had dementia means that I prioritise keeping my brain healthy. I don't neglect other aspects of my health, but I keep my brain front of mind, as it were!

We might inherit genetic variations that predispose us to specific diseases, or we might be lucky and receive gene variants that deliver disease resistance. Our own family histories can help to identify the genetic hand that we've been dealt.

Your ancestral health portrait

You're going to create a very specific family tree. This one will look at the illnesses, longevity and causes of death of family members. On the next page you'll find an outline to fill in.

- Gather as much information as you can about the health of family members. Talk to other relatives about your family. Your older cousin might recall that (great-) granny had arthritis, even if you're too young to remember.
- Has anyone in your family undertaken a genealogy project? They might have collected death certificates or health records as evidence. Ask them to share these with you.
- Include those who are still alive, particularly parents and uncles/aunts. List any illnesses or chronic conditions that they might have and add their current age.
- For family members who are no longer alive, add the cause of death, their age when they died and any health issues you're aware of.

When I did mine, I realised that there is dementia on both sides of my family, and some very long-lived women who didn't spend their final years in good health. It was another reminder that health span (the number of healthy years we can look forward to) is more important than lifespan. It's a great tool in helping me stick to my own age-well plan.

Your ancestral health portrait to fill out

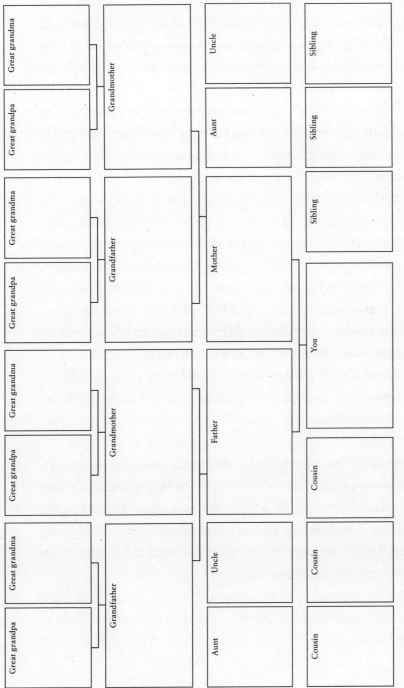

Add:
- Current age or age when they died
- Cause of death
- Other known conditions

Should you have a genetic test?

If you want to explore your genetic inheritance further, you might consider a genetic test. This will review a fraction of your genes and give you an outline of some health issues to factor into your age-well plan.

For the Age-Well Project both my co-author, Annabel, and I had our genes analysed by an American company called 23andme (23andme.com). We ordered kits online, spat into test tubes and waited for the results.

Annabel was incredibly enthusiastic about the whole process; I was terrified.

What I dreaded most was a result revealing that I carry the ApoE4 gene, which is linked to increased Alzheimer's risk. We all inherit one ApoE gene from each parent. The big question is: what number is it? ApoE2, the least common, seems to reduce the risk of Alzheimer's; ApoE3 – the most common – makes no difference; but ApoE4 is the one to be concerned about. Carrying one ApoE4 gene doubles the risk of Alzheimer's; carrying two quadruples it. The test revealed that I, in common with about 25 per cent of the population, carry one ApoE4 gene.

Once I had the results, and looked at the stats, I was strangely comforted. My genetic risk of developing Alzheimer's is 14 per cent between the ages of 65 and 80, and one in three over the age of 80. That's pretty high, but considering that I would have put my risk factor near to 100 per cent before I did the test, the results were an enormous relief.

Getting a genetic test is a personal choice. If you're curious, research it well and get the best one you can afford. Bear in mind the words of Professor Helen Stokes-Lampard, chair of the Royal College of GPs, who has said that genetic testing should 'never be taken lightly'. She explained, 'Many things that will be picked up by genetic testing will be unimportant or of dubious value, and these could leave people unnecessarily confused and distressed.'

You'll also need to run your results through a secondary service – try Promethease, Genomelink or foundmyfitness.com – to extract all the health information available in your raw data. Most services charge a small fee for this, about $10–$20.

Be aware that any company that tests your genes will ask you to sign a waiver allowing them to store your data. I took the view that my data might help health researchers in the future, and I tried not to worry about it. If you are concerned about data protection, and how the information might be used, read the small print very carefully.

Always remember that lifestyle has a huge impact on how our genes are expressed, and much of our genetic inheritance can be modified by how we eat, move and live. We'll be exploring all those factors in the weeks to come.

The Top 10: your own health portrait

Just as you have created an ancestral health portrait, you need to put together a portrait of yourself, but don't worry – no drawing required! You do need to get to grips with the Top 10 key facts and figures about yourself, take ownership of them and commit to tracking them from now onwards. Taking control of your own health as you age means knowing your numbers. Even if all your results are fantastically healthy, keep a note of the results as a baseline for the future.

In Appendix 1 (page 237) you'll find tables detailing what your numbers should be to stay within a healthy range. These are based on NHS guidelines unless otherwise stated.

1 Weight

This isn't a diet book, but recording your weight now is a good way to keep track of it. It's not nearly as important as your body mass index (BMI) or waist-to-hip ratio, but it's worth knowing at this point.

Your weight:

Date of test:

2 Body mass index (BMI)

Research shows that obesity in mid- to late life increases the risk of dementia, type-2 diabetes, high blood pressure, some cancers and cardiovascular disease. At the other end of the scale (literally) being underweight increases a woman's risk of osteoporosis and anaemia. Underweight people over 80 are more likely to die than those who have a normal weight. Body Mass Index (BMI) refers to the ratio between your height and your weight.

How to test: you can work this out yourself. For most adults, an ideal BMI is in the 18.5 to 24.9 range. Work out your height in metres squared. If you're 1m 60cm tall, that's $1.6 \times 1.6 = 2.56$. Now divide your weight in kilos by this figure. The result is your BMI. The NHS website, www.nhs.uk, has a BMI calculator that does the maths for you and offers advice.

Your result:

Date of test:

3 Waist-to-hip ratio

This is a good indicator of abdominal fat, which even thin people can carry in dangerous quantities. Carrying fat around our internal organs increases the risk of cardiovascular disease, diabetes and heart attacks. Unhealthy waist-to-hip ratios can predict cardiovascular disease better than Body Mass Index.

How to test: you can work this out yourself, too. Measure your waist in centimetres just above the navel, and then measure your hips at their widest point. Now divide your waist measurement by your hip measurement. According to the WHO, the ideal result for women is below 0.85 and for men below 1.00.

Your result:

Date of test:

4 Blood pressure

Our blood pressure can rise without us knowing as we age and needs to be tested at least every two years. If your pressure is high or borderline high (that is, systolic blood pressure between 120 and 139, and diastolic blood pressure between 80 and 89), check it at least once a year, or more often if your doctor suggests it.

High blood pressure is linked to an increased risk of stroke, heart attack, Alzheimer's disease and vascular dementia. From the age of 30 our blood vessels stiffen and narrow, so their walls are thicker, which in turn leads to higher pressure. By the age of 65, 50 per cent of us will have high blood pressure, known as hypertension.

Where to get tested: your doctor's surgery or a local pharmacy (ask if yours offers a blood pressure service).

Your result:

Date of test:

5 Resting heart rate

A lower resting heart rate implies more efficient heart function and better cardiovascular fitness. A stronger and more efficient heart pumps more blood each time it contracts, needing fewer beats per minute to do its job. A resting heart rate can be anything between 60 and 100 beats per minute.

Where to get tested: at your doctor's surgery or a gym. You can take your own pulse, but make sure that you have been resting for at least five minutes before you check it.

Your result:

Date of test:

6 Cholesterol levels

Your cholesterol levels should be checked every five years. We used to think that all cholesterol is bad, but in fact it's vital for many processes within the body and brain. When you get tested, ask your doctor for a full lipid profile. This will cover both LDL (low-density lipoprotein) and HDL (high-density lipoprotein). LDL is known as 'bad' cholesterol and forms hard plaques in the arteries, elevating heart attack risk. HDL is referred to as 'good' cholesterol as it clears the build-up of LDL, transporting it back to the liver for recycling or excretion. A full lipid profile will also test triglyceride levels. Triglycerides are a form of fat the body uses for energy: too many of them circulating in our blood can also contribute to heart disease.

Where to get tested: at your doctor's surgery, pharmacist or NHS Health Check.

Your result:

Date of test:

7 Blood glucose levels

Elevated blood sugar is the greatest risk for diabetes and is the result of the body's failure to respond to insulin. The number of people in the UK with type-2 diabetes has doubled in the last 20 years, and it's estimated that there are around half a million undiagnosed cases in this country alone. Risk factors include being overweight, a sedentary lifestyle, high blood pressure and high cholesterol levels.

Where to get tested: at your doctor's surgery or NHS Health Check.

Your result:

Date of test:

8 Vitamin D levels

Pretty much everyone in the UK has insufficient vitamin D, which is vital for respiratory, bone, brain and heart health, as well as immune function. Research published during the coronavirus epidemic revealed that people who are deficient in vitamin D are at increased risk of Covid-19. It's worth having your levels checked while you are having other tests, and taking a supplement. Commit to supplementing from October until May if you get out in the sun in the summer, or all year round if you don't. If you have broader concerns about vitamin and mineral deficiencies, consider asking for a complete blood count.

Where to get tested: at your doctor's surgery or NHS Health Check.

Your result:

Date of test:

9 DEXA/bone density scan

If you're at risk of osteoporosis, or have a history of broken bones, your doctor might want to send you for a DEXA scan. I was offered one automatically when I broke my wrist five years ago.

Where to get tested: at your doctor's surgery or NHS Health Check.

Your result:

Date of test:

10 C-reactive protein test

The C-reactive protein test measures the amount of inflammation in your body. It's not essential, but it might be worth considering if you have a family history of inflammatory diseases.

Where to get tested: ask your GP.

Your result:

Date of test:

Congratulations! You have made a great start on your health portrait. Make sure you keep a record of these numbers in the years to come and record any changes.

Talk to your GP

If you have any worrying results, discuss them with your GP. Get advice from them on how best to tackle any health issues that might have been highlighted. Also, make sure that you are up to date with mammograms, smears, colonoscopies and any other tests offered by the NHS to those in your age range.

Blue Zoners and SuperAgers

I'd like to introduce you to some very special people who can teach us a lot about ageing well.

Blue Zoners live in areas of the world with the highest concentration of centenarians. Five of these Blue Zones have been identified across the world: Okinawa in Japan, Loma Linda in California, the Greek island of Ikaria, the Barbàgia region of Sardinia and the Nicoya Peninsula in Costa Rica. In each location, a cluster of lifestyle traits have led to exceptionally long-lived populations:

- A sense of purpose
- Little stress
- A Mediterranean diet with lots of beans, whole grains, vegetables and a little wine
- Eating until 80 per cent full (see page 66)
- A sense of community and respect for elders
- Natural movement throughout the day, roughly every 20 minutes or so
- Focusing on family and close friendships
- A spiritual practice

How many of those can you tick off? You can learn more about Blue Zones at www.bluezones.com.

SuperAgers is the term used to refer to those amazing older people whom you might know or have heard about. The ones who are still working into their eighties and nineties, or competing in sporting events, or who are extremely mentally agile despite their advancing years. They are less likely to suffer from dementia, and more likely to live to 100, than the rest of us. Of course, every SuperAger is different, but researchers have identified some common traits:[14]

- Staying physically active
- Continuing to challenge themselves mentally
- Strong social connections
- More neurons in the part of the brain linked to attention and working memory
- Resilience to life's ups and downs, and more 'grit'
- More extroverted and less neurotic

Your personal age-well plan – purpose and portraits

Review what you have achieved this week. You have:

- Set out your purpose in ageing well.
- Learnt about the science of ageing and how you can make a difference to how you age.
- Reviewed the external ageing factors you're most concerned about.
- Created two portraits: one of your family health history and one of your own health.

Based on this, what are the key areas that you need to focus on in your age-well plan?

Tick below or note down the areas you need to prioritise. Which of the external risk factors do you need to focus on most?

- ☐ Smoking
- ☐ Bad diet
- ☐ Excess weight
- ☐ Sedentary behaviour
- ☐ Stress
- ☐ Lack of sleep
- ☐ Over-consumption of alcohol
- ☐ Air pollution
- ☐ Toxins and plastics
- ☐ Loneliness

Does your ancestral health portrait reveal any patterns or cause for concern? Note them here:

Have you considered having a genetic test and weighed up the pros and cons?

Does your personal health portrait reveal any areas you need to focus on? Talk to your doctor about how you're going to tackle them. All the issues listed here will benefit from the age-well protocols you're going to work on in the coming weeks.

- ☐ Weight
- ☐ BMI
- ☐ Waist-to-hip ratio

☐   Blood pressure
☐   Resting heart rate
☐   Cholesterol levels
☐   Blood glucose
☐   Vitamin D level
☐   DEXA/bone density scan (if necessary)
☐   C-reactive protein test (if necessary)

Set your intentions – plan ahead

Where will you focus as you start your age-well plan?

Based on the tick list you have just completed, write out your intentions for your own age-well plan. Perhaps your life is very sedentary, or you can see a strong family history of cardiovascular disease, or your waist-to-hip ratio needs attention. Use this information to help you personalise elements of your plan and focus on the changes you make over the coming weeks. For example, *In the next six weeks I will review my sleep habits, reduce my exposure to pollution and work to lower my blood pressure.*

It might feel strange to write this out, but the act of setting down our intentions makes us more likely to stick to them. Remember that this is where you commit to ageing well.

In the next six weeks I will ...

Finally, write out your age-well purpose again here to help you remember it:

DR STEPHAN RECHTSCHAFFEN OF BLUE SPIRIT, COSTA RICA

'Have a plan – age well for life'

Dr Stephan Rechtschaffen is an integrative physician, best-selling author and founder of the world-renowned Omega Institute in New York State and the Blue Spirit Retreat Centre in Nosara, Costa Rica.

Stephan lives and works on a verdant hillside overlooking the crystal-clear seas that lap the Nicoya Peninsula, Costa Rica. It's a picture-perfect location to build a wellness retreat, and happens to be one of the world's Blue Zones (see page 38). Stephan discovered the spot after establishing a holistic health centre, the Omega Institute, in the United States. 'It wasn't until I was here that I found out about the Blue Zones and [Blue Zones researcher] Dan Buettner's work – which I think is very interesting – but I wanted to take it further,' he explains.

At Blue Spirit, he's created a Longevity Centre to treat key drivers of the chronic diseases of ageing: inflammation, heavy metal toxicity, mitochondrial function and oxidative stress. The centre offers antioxidant infusions, heavy metal testing and a 'gym' for mitochondria. The health of these 'batteries', which provide our cells with energy, is the focus of Stephan's work. 'Nutrients go into the cell, and energy, in a form known as ATP, comes out. It's like going to the ATM and getting dollars. The downside is that, like a car burning gas, there's always a toxic by-product, which, in the body, produces oxidative stress. We want the fuel-burning process to be as efficient as possible and to produce as much energy as it can. If you keep your mitochondria healthy, then you won't age as fast. The ageing of your mitochondria *is* your ageing.'

At 72, Stephan is lean, trim and full of energy. He's a firm believer in intermittent fasting, ordering a soya milk cappuccino when we meet mid-morning, but otherwise not breaking his fast until lunchtime. 'I have a big lunch, but when I go to dinner I'm always amazed that people will have an appetiser, a main and a dessert. I maybe have two appetisers: it's really light eating.' He focuses his diet on organic vegetables and hasn't eaten meat for 50 years, although he's not averse to eating fish.

Stephan plays tennis four or five times a week and does Pilates twice a week. But physical exercise is only part of the story – there needs to be time for contemplation too. 'Healthy longevity stems from within. It's not some outer thing, just lifting weights or eating right; so many other elements play a role as well,' he explains. He believes that, as we get older, we need to allow our bodies to rest, restore and repair, factors that are often overlooked in a world that demands we are always in 'on' mode. He aims to sleep seven hours a night and believes that good mental health is as critical to ageing well as good physical health.

'Despite all the problems in the world, how do we live in good mood?' he asks. 'The Dalai Lama has seen the people of his country tortured and killed, and he cares deeply about it, but he maintains good mood.' Stephan has a deep daily meditation practice and believes that true well-being and living a meaningful life depend to a large degree on our state of mind. 'It's about finding happiness. In that regard, I consider myself very privileged: I get to live in a beautiful place, work with amazing people and help others.'

You can read more at bluespiritcostarica.com

WEEK 2

How to Eat

Eating to age well isn't about faddy diets. I'm not going to suggest you give up a food group, or go vegan, or ketotarian, or Paleo, or pegan or any of those other strange-sounding regimes. All of them have passionate adherents and, if that's your thing, go for it. But eating for longevity is about balance, moderation and adaptability. What I'm going to suggest is sensible, doable and based on decades of research. Oh, and it's delicious too.

Eat well, age well

My age-well journey began in the kitchen, which is why I suggest you start there too. I had to relearn *how* and *what* to eat. This week you'll consider your own nutrition and how you can reframe it as part of your age-well plan. By the end of the week you'll be on track for a lifetime of eating for healthy longevity by making simple shifts in your diet. One week to change your diet may seem intense but remember you'll be practising and evolving it in the weeks to come.

What we eat isn't just fuel for our bodies; it also impacts our immune system and longevity pathways, influencing how we age at the most basic, cellular level. This week you'll examine the world's best-researched diet and start cooking it yourself, you'll junk the junk and say 'so long, sugar', you'll look at the power of vegetables and how to work them into your diet all day, every day, and you'll be good to your gut, getting your microbiota (the trillions of bacteria, viruses and fungi which live in our intestines) working to help you age well. You'll start fasting, which is probably the simplest way to fire up the body's resources and get it working to repair our ageing cells. Don't panic at the word 'fasting' (I know I did); there's a way to do it so that you'll barely notice – trust me.

In Appendix II, you'll find a complete one-week menu plan with recipes and ideas to get you eating the age-well way. It's the way I cook, and eat, every day. I've found being in control of what I consume each day tremendously empowering, and I hope you will, too. It helps me to stay focused on my age-well plan *and* – the really good news – I feel better than ever right now.

A word about weight loss

This isn't a diet book, but the reality is that in the UK 78 per cent of men and over two-thirds of women aged 45–74 are overweight or obese.[1]

You know your BMI and waist-to-hip ratio now, and how those numbers might impact your longevity. The way of eating you're going to focus on this week delivers age-well benefits and can be adapted for weight loss if that's what you need.

Researchers have found that a 5 per cent weight loss is enough to make a dramatic difference to obese patients' risk for diabetes and cardiovascular disease, two of the most prevalent chronic conditions of ageing.[2] Being overweight also affects immune function: the Covid-19 pandemic disproportionately affected older people who were overweight when they contracted the virus. One small study found that three-quarters of people admitted to intensive care units were obese.[3]

When I started my own age-well plan, I lost weight, and it has remained stable ever since. I don't count calories or follow a restricted diet. I kicked out processed foods, cut right down on sugar and started to fast overnight. I'll explain how in the coming pages. Understanding the science of longevity, and knowing my purpose in ageing well, keeps me motivated.

Assess yourself as you start the week

The questions overleaf are based on the Mediterranean Diet Adherence Screener, which is widely used to assess dietary quality.

I've tweaked it to include longevity-specific research to help you build your own age-well diet plan. There's no ideal starting point, so don't worry if you answer 'no' to every question. The important thing is, as always, that you're starting now. After seven days your answers will be different.

Questionnaire: diet – what are you eating now?

		Yes	No
1	Do you use olive oil as your main culinary fat?	☐	☐
2	Do you consume at least five 80g portions of vegetables each day?	☐	☐
3	Do you eat fewer than seven portions of meat each week?	☐	☐
4	Do you drink seven or fewer units of alcohol each week?	☐	☐
5	Do you eat at least three portions of beans/pulses each week?	☐	☐
6	Do you eat at least two portions of oily fish each week?	☐	☐
7	Do you consume commercially made sweets, cakes or ice cream fewer than three times a week?	☐	☐
8	Do you eat at least two 30g servings of nuts each week?	☐	☐
9	Do you eat at least 25g of fibre each day? (See page 81 to calculate your fibre intake.)	☐	☐
10	Do you fast overnight for 12–14 hours?	☐	☐

Your score:

If you had plenty of 'yes' answers, congratulations! You're well on your way to eating the age-well way. Lots of 'no' answers? Let's start making some simple changes.

By the end of this week you will:

- Have a clearer path to weight loss, if you need it.
- Understand the importance of home cooking and how to find time to do it.
- Eat a more Mediterranean-style diet and understand its impact on your health.
- Work green leafy vegetables and/or berries into every meal.
- Focus on good gut health.
- Fast – and find the best way for you to work this into your life.
- Calculate your fibre intake and get at least 25g a day.
- Cut heavily processed foods from your diet and focus on whole foods.
- Reduce your sugar intake.
- Have re-evaluated your relationship with alcohol.
- Stay properly hydrated and use coffee and tea to help you age well.
- Enjoy plant proteins and eat less meat.

The big picture: diet – 5 essential lessons

Many, many books and academic reports have been written on ageing and diet. I'm going to keep it really simple and highlight the five most important actions you can take, beginning today and continuing for the rest of your life. In the Top 10 section you'll discover simple ways to make them work in your life every day.

1 Junk the junk

Familiarise yourself with the term 'ultra-processed foods' (UPFs). This refers to the vast majority of pre-prepared foods chock-full of ingredients that you won't have in your kitchen at home: emulsifiers, corn syrups, protein isolates ... I could write a very long list. Some of them are ostensibly healthy – vegan sausages, lentil puffs, almond milk – but they've been constructed in such a way that they bear very little resemblance to the original ingredients. Over 50 per cent of calories consumed in the UK come from these foods.

If one of your goals for your age-well plan is to lose weight, cutting out these UPFs will make a huge difference. When I needed to lose weight, they were the first thing that had to go. Not only are they often laden with sugars and fats, their chemical make-up prevents our satiety mechanism from kicking in. Which is why it's possible to eat an entire box of Jaffa Cakes or a family pack of crisps (we've all done it) and be hungry again almost straight away.

Recent research shows that when people eat a diet of UPFs they not only consume more calories and gain weight, but also their appetite-suppressing hormones decrease and their hunger hormones increase.[4] In a month-long experiment, volunteers ate ultra-processed foods for two weeks, and healthy, unprocessed foods for two weeks. The two regimes were matched for calorific content as well as levels of sugar, fat, protein and fibre. The participants could eat as much or as little as they wanted. During the weeks they were eating UPFs, they put on at least 1kg (2lb) each, consumed 500 calories a day more, and their hunger hormones failed to switch off.

Eating a diet overly reliant on processed foods has also been linked to impaired immune response and an increased risk of heart attack, stroke, diabetes and early death.[5] People who eat too much sugar, salt and processed foods, rather than whole grains, vegetables and fruit, have shorter telomeres. It's not just about carrying a few extra pounds or a bit of a spare tyre, the food we eat fuels the ageing process at a cellular level. It's about choosing the whole apple over the apple juice, a bowl of porridge over a granola bar and unprocessed meat over bacon. (Sorry about the bacon.)

A note on salt

Consuming too much salt is linked to high blood pressure. Ultra-processed foods are often high in salt, although levels are being reduced in the UK. Eating unprocessed foods dramatically reduces our salt intake. When I cook I use small amounts of sea salt and liberal quantities of both herbs and spices to add flavour. The recommended daily intake of salt in the UK is 6g (about one teaspoon of table salt). Be guided by your doctor if you have concerns about your salt intake.

---

2 Make it fast

In Week 1 you learnt about the process of autophagy (page 22), when our body chomps through cellular waste products, broken DNA and damaged proteins. As we age, the process slows down and our bodies are overwhelmed by all this biological gunk, making us frail and chronically sick. Wouldn't it be great if we could kick-start autophagy and clear out the rubbish? Luckily, we can, but it does mean getting a bit hungry.[6]

To quote Harvard researcher and author of *Lifespan: Why We Age and Why We Don't Have To*, David Sinclair, 'After twenty-five years of researching ageing and having read thousands of scientific papers, if there is ... one sure-fire way to stay healthy longer ... it's this: eat less.'

Hundreds of studies have shown that restricting the calorific intake of mice, rats and fruit flies extends their lives. A long-term study of rhesus monkeys fed 30 per cent fewer calories found they could live up to 40 years,[7] which equates to about 120 for humans.

It's rather harder for us to stick to a reduced-calorie diet for decades, however compelling the longevity benefits. We're simply not used to being hungry any more, although our ancestors were used to a cycle of feast and famine as they hunted on the savannah. Food is so freely available to us now that we've lost touch with what it feels like to be famished.

It seems there's a shortcut that brings us the benefits of calorie restriction without the ever-present hunger, however. It's known as intermittent fasting: going without food for a short(ish) period of time and then eating normally. Fasting gives the body time to use up the glucose stored in the liver, then to switch to energy production from stored fat. This energy source is known as ketones, or ketone bodies. When the body is in this state, inflammation levels drop, while autophagy, sirtuin and telomere activity increase: exactly the age-well benefits we want.

3 Make it Medi

The principles of the Mediterranean diet lie at the heart of the age-well plan.

The first thing to know is that it's not a 'diet' – it's a way of life. The term refers to the traditional mode of eating in southern European countries, where incidences of heart disease, cancer, diabetes and dementia are all lower than they are in the UK and US. It's a diet that has grown out of poverty and lack, where processed food, sugar and meat were too expensive to consume regularly or simply unavailable.

'Mediterranean diet' has become shorthand for a way of eating that emphasises pulses, beans, vegetables, olive oil, fermented dairy, whole grains, fish, herbs and spices, nuts and berries, red wine and a little meat. If this represents a big change in the way you eat now, take it slowly. Pick a recipe from the age-well menu plan (Appendix III, page 243) and give it a go, then try another one. Plan your meals in advance so that you can check how many of these ingredients you're integrating into your diet as you go.

Why does it work? It seems that the diet slows the ageing process by reducing damage to our telomeres.[8] These are the protective shoelace-tip-like caps on the ends of your chromosomes that you learnt about in Week 1. Shortened telomeres are considered a hallmark of ageing, but the Medi diet can keep them long and help them to replenish themselves.

The result is that the Mediterranean diet has been linked to a reduction in almost all the chronic conditions of ageing, and a lower risk of death overall.[9] Recent research (on women) links the diet with a one-quarter lower risk of cardiovascular disease.

To put that into context, it's the same risk reduction as that conferred by taking statins, which are regularly prescribed to lower cardiovascular risk.[10] And it's also been linked to better brain function in older adults.[11]

The Medi diet might be the recipe for a long and happy life, but it doesn't come out of a packet. I keep it ultra-simple though: a piece of grilled fish, loads of vegetables, a handful of nuts, plenty of pulses and a cheeky glass of red wine!

4 Pick up plants

I'm not vegan or vegetarian, but creating my own age-well plan has meant eating a whole lot more plants. Vegetables, pulses and whole grains are the mainstays of my diet these days. By filling my plate with plant-based whole foods, I'm able to crowd out meat, dairy and processed foods – not completely, but the balance has very definitely shifted.

I focus on plant-based protein sources – beans, pulses and pseudo-cereals such as quinoa. All proteins are made up of smaller building blocks called amino acids, linked together in chains. Animal protein sources – meat, dairy and eggs – contain all the amino acids that our bodies need. They're a one-stop shop, as it were, for our protein needs. Plant-based proteins don't provide the full complement of amino acids in one go, so our bodies have to work a little harder to build the amino acid chains we need. But this can be a good thing for longevity.

In Week 1 we learnt about the biological decline that happens as we age, and how our body's repair mechanisms can go awry. And we learnt that the signalling systems in our bodies decode energy and nutrient levels before sending operating instructions to our cells. When there are plenty of amino acids in the body, our signalling systems know that times are good.[12] They send out the signal to 'Grow! Grow! Grow!' But, as we age, we want our cells to get the message 'Repair! Repair! Repair!' We need enough amino acids from protein to keep our muscles and immune systems strong, approximately 1 gram of protein per kilo of body weight, but the focus should be on keeping DNA in a good state of repair.

The other great benefit vegetables gift to our longevity is that they help to combat the oxidative stress (page 23) that accumulates in our bodies as we age. Plants have complex chemistry to protect them from predators and harsh conditions. Put simply, when we consume plants, we benefit from those phytonutrients, too; for example, folate found in green vegetables helps to keep our telomeres long and has a positive impact on cognition in older adults. Quercetin, found in apples, onions and buckwheat, helps to fight inflammation and kick-starts sirtuins to manage those zombie senescent cells (page 23);[13] and anthocyanins (the deep blues and purples that give blueberries their colour) protect the lining of our arteries. Every vegetable has a similar story: they're our best allies in the fight to age well.

5 Be good to your gut

Our bodies are home to a universe of microbes. Some flourish on our skin, but the vast majority take up residence in our digestive tract.

They impact a huge range of processes, from how we digest food to our mood and immune responses. Our microbial cells outnumber our human cells by ten to one: that's mind-blowing. We are essentially hosts to a teeming world we never see, which (should) work in harmony with our bodies. These trillions of guests are a delicate balance of good and bad, depending on how they impact on our health. Unfortunately, our modern, Western diet feeds the bad microbiota and, just as importantly, starves the good. The bad bacteria tend to feed on sugar and unhealthy fats, the good on unprocessed plants with a high fibre content.

The end result is that the modern-day microbiome has become sparse compared to that of our ancestors: our diets lack the variety of foods and fibre they consumed. Add to that the natural depletion that comes with age and many of us are faced with a sub-par microbiome.

The inflammation you learnt about in Week 1 also has an impact on your gut microbiota. And a reduced microbiome may in return play a role in inflammation – creating a vicious cycle. Gut microbiota imbalances become both the causes and the effects of the inflamm-ageing process.[14] The alteration of our microbiota as we age is so marked that researchers are able to use samples of gut bacteria to predict a person's age within four years.[15]

Pick almost any of the chronic diseases of ageing – obesity, type-2 diabetes, some cancers, heart disease – and there's research indicating that an imbalance (dysbiosis) in the microbiome may be one of the causes. The link between gut and brain is particularly powerful: scientists refer to the gut as our 'second brain'. Messages pass from the gut to the brain, and back again, via the gut–brain axis, and particular strains of bad gut microbiota have been linked to Alzheimer's disease, Parkinson's and depression. Improving the quality of the bacteria in our gut will help us age well.

How I make it work – cooking

When I say that my age-well plan began in the kitchen, I do mean by actually *cooking*. There's no way round it, cooking our own food allows us to take responsibility for our diet and our health. I'm not talking about elaborate, gourmet cooking, but simple dishes that you and your family will enjoy. By preparing food ourselves, we can choose healthful, longevity-inducing ingredients as well as controlling levels of sugar, salt and fat.

This does take more time than bunging a ready meal in the microwave, of course, but I've learnt to prioritise and take short-cuts. Have a look at the menu plan in Appendix III. Age-well breakfast pots can be prepared the night before you need them; I almost always have prepped greens stashed in the fridge to add leafy goodness to a meal, and tinned beans can transform into protein-rich main courses, such as Black Bean Chilli and Sweet Potato Tacos (page 252), in minutes. My freezer is my friend when it comes to bigger batches of soups, stews and chillies that I can pull out at the last minute.

Cooking to age well has meant more, but smaller, dishes on the table. I've said goodbye to meat-and-two-veg eating and put plants front and centre. Again, that doesn't mean lots more work: it could be a bowl of beautiful tomatoes or a lentil salad that lasts for a few days. I've learnt to plan and prep in advance so that I know what my family and I will be eating each day, and I'm not spending time repeatedly running to the shops. And, most importantly, I know how good I feel after eating this way.

My age-well mantra

Prep and plan! I chop vegetables ready for the evening while my daughter's eating breakfast, write a weekly menu so that I'm not flailing around wondering what's for dinner, and use downtime on a Sunday to make a bean-based dish to eat later in the week.

The Top 10: eat to age well every day

Eating well to age well involves small shifts in your day-to-day life, gently moving the dial on what you consume for breakfast, lunch and dinner. There's a one-week menu plan in Appendix III, but this isn't a quick-fix-lose-seven-pounds-in-seven-days kind of diet. It's a way of eating that will stay with you for the rest of your life. Below are ten simple things to do every day. I've given suggestions for making each one work in your life – tick these off so that you can track your progress. If it seems over-whelming, just pick one doable action and start with that. When you've nailed it, pick another. You've got this! Write down any concerns, ideas or notes underneath each section.

1 Go for green leafy vegetables

If you do nothing else on your age-well plan, eat more green leafy vegetables. These nutritional powerhouses have been linked to better eye, heart and liver health, as well as reduced diabetes risk and slower cognitive decline. (If you have thyroid issues, talk to your doctor about your intake of greens.)

☐ Work them into breakfast, lunch and dinner. I make sure I have greens in two meals a day. See the menu plan at the end of the book for inspiration.

☐ Focus on cruciferous vegetables (i.e. brassicas). Broccoli, cabbage, cauliflower, pak choi, kale and Brussels sprouts are all rich sources of a compound called sulforaphane, which regulates a key longevity pathway that protects us from oxidative stress.

☐ Always grab at least one bag or bunch of greens (those listed above but also baby spinach, chard, cavolo nero – anything goes) each time you go to the supermarket or greengrocer. I hate food waste, so I always make sure I use them up!

☐ Steam, blanch, sauté, stir-fry or even roast. There are myriad ways to cook your veg. Just promise me that you won't overcook them. A couple of minutes is usually enough, unless you're roasting them.

☐ Pep up greens with a sprinkling of salt, a squeeze of lemon, a pinch of chilli, a scattering of toasted nuts.

2 Eat brightly coloured vegetables

Some of the most beautiful fruits and vegetables are also the ones that are best for us. The vibrant colours that attract our eyes are the source of antioxidants, plus vitamins C and A, which help us to thrive, supporting immune function and quelling inflammation.

☐ Eat the rainbow – the more of those beautiful colours we consume, the better. How many colours can you get onto your plate in one day?

☐ Don't just think of vegetables as a side dish – make them the main event. Freestyle with the plant-based recipes in the menu plan and add your own extras.

☐ Make dishes that you can mix and match across a couple of days – having a few different meals that I can pull out of the fridge quickly is a godsend. You'll find beetroot hummus, roast vegetables, quick pickles and crudités in my fridge on a regular basis.

☐ Make the most of sweet vegetables and you won't notice that you're eating less sugar: sweet potatoes, squash and peppers all have a natural sweetness but are also packed with fibre and polyphenols (antioxidants which protect the body from free radicals – see page 23). Roasting brings out the taste.

3 Fill up on fibre

When researchers crunched down almost 40 years' worth of research into the health benefits of fibre, they found it was linked to a 15–30 per cent decrease in death from heart disease and all other causes. Our gut microbiota ferment fibre to create short-chain fatty acids, which help the body fight inflammation, protect the brain and regulate the immune system.

☐ Aim for 25–29g of fibre a day. While we were writing *The Age-Well Project* I kept a fibre diary to make sure that I was on track, and I urge you to do the same this week. There's a Fibre Tracker on page 82 and a rundown of the fibre content of the best age-well foods on page 81.

☐ If you're eating more fibre, drink more water, too. You need to keep things moving, as it were.

☐ Experiment with fibre-packed whole grains. I love the unusual ones such as freekeh, farro and amaranth. Hunt them down in health-food shops and work them into your daily diet. Use them to replace rice or pasta in your cooking.

☐ Think about where the fibre's coming from in each meal as you plan.

4 Control the carbs, especially if you're trying to lose weight

For decades, governmental health advice urged us to fill up on carbohydrates while limiting our intake of protein and fats. Now this advice has been implicated in growing rates of obesity and diabetes across the Western world. Eating too many carbohydrates, particularly processed sugars and flours, spikes insulin levels, leading to weight gain and inflammation.

☐ Keep carbohydrates whole grain and the portions small. Think about carb quality (the nutrients it delivers) rather than quantity. Make sure your carbs are delivering plenty of fibre, as above.

☐ Crowd out refined carbohydrates such as white flour and white rice with plenty of vegetables, which are more nutritionally dense.

☐ No more than one-quarter of your plate should be wholegrain carbs, one-quarter protein and half vegetables, particularly if you are trying to lose a few pounds.

☐ Look online for Canada's food guide (food-guide. canada.ca/en). It's a clear visual representation of the plate described above. Canada is the first country in the world to publish guidelines that put the emphasis firmly on eating lots of vegetables.

5 Fast overnight

There are many different ways to fast. You might have heard of the 5:2 diet, which works by restricting calories to 500 a day for women and 600 a day for men, two days a week. Dr Valter Longo, author of *The Longevity Diet*, suggests a low-calorie fast for five days, up to once a month. But it seems a consensus is forming among experts that overnight fasting is the simplest way to gain the health benefits of fasting without too much hunger.

☐ An easy way to try an overnight fast is 12 hours' fasting, and a 12-hour eating window (you have all your meals within 12 hours). If you finish dinner by 8pm, have breakfast at 8am.

☐ When you feel comfortable with that, try to extend your fasting window a little further. The 16:8 intermittent fast (16 hours' fasting, eight-hours eating window) is popular.

☐ I get a bit too hungry on 16:8, particularly when I'm at work. I aim for a sweet spot of a 14-hour fast, 10-hour eating window. I aim to finish dinner by 8.30pm and have breakfast at 10.30–11am. I've come to see breakfast as a mid-morning activity, not the start to my day. This 10-hour eating window has also been found to benefit people with metabolic syndrome (the precursor to dia-betes). If you are insulin-resistant or have diabetes, talk to your doctor before fasting.

☐ Keep hydrated during your fast: I have lemon water first thing, black coffee or tea with a splash of milk around 9am and take an age-well breakfast pot to work to eat mid-morning.

6 Berries are best

The beautiful, jewel-like colours of berries come from antho-cyanins, a source of antioxidants. They reduce oxidative stress and inflammation in the body as we age. Berries have also been linked to increased plasticity in the brain, helping neurons (nerve cells) to form new connections and boosting memory.[16] They're high in fibre, with very little sugar, making them my go-to fruit each day.

☐ Just as two portions of leafy greens are non-negotiable in my day, so is a portion of berries. If I don't have berries with my breakfast, I make sure to eat them with some yogurt or kefir as a dessert, or just grab a handful as a snack (usually with a few nuts, too, to help me feel full).

☐ Blueberries, raspberries, cranberries, mulberries and strawberries are all good. Mix them up and buy what's in season. I particularly love blackberry picking in early autumn – there's something very satisfying about forag-ing for wild food.

☐ I freeze my foraged blackberries and dig into them throughout the year. I also buy frozen blueberries and raspberries when they're out of season.

☐ I throw frozen berries into my breakfast pots, porridge and smoothies every day.

My age-well mantra

Berries, greens, greens! Every. Single. Day.

7 Feed your gut

The trillions of guests we welcome into our digestive tracts need to eat well to thrive. And for this gut-based throng, eating well means a steady supply of probiotics and prebiotics from high-fibre plants and fermented foods.

☐ You've probably heard of *probiotics* – they increase the quantity of good bacteria in our gut and help support immunity. The best sources are fermented foods – traditional vegetable ferments such as sauerkraut and kimchi, and fermented dairy such as kefir and natural live yogurt. A tablespoon or two a day is enough, as overdoing it can cause dysbiosis.

☐ *Prebiotics* provide nourishment for our microbiota, literally feeding our gut. Good sources of prebiotics include leeks, onions, garlic, bananas, asparagus, apples, oats, pulses and whole grains.

☐ Don't just eat for gut health, drink for it too. Kombucha (fermented tea) is a delicious source of probiotics – bonus points if you make your own – and coffee drinkers have a greater abundance of anti-inflammatory bacteria in their guts.

☐ Gut happiness comes not just from what you consume, but also what you don't. Fasting appears to give gut microbiota the opportunity to regenerate gut stem cells, balance out good and bad bacteria and increase bacterial diversity.

8 Drink water, tea, coffee

Staying properly hydrated, and reaping the benefits of coffee and tea each day, is key to ageing well. As we age, our water reserves decline due to a reduction in muscle mass, our kidneys become less effective at retaining water, and hormonal signals that trigger thirst become blunted.[17] Recent research links drinking green tea to an extra 19 months of healthy life expectancy, probably due to its high polyphenol (plant antioxidants) content. Coffee is a longevity superstar – as well as boosting gut health, its polyphenols combat cell damage, boost insulin sensitivity and decrease blood pressure.

☐ Drink filtered water all day, every day. Start with a simple filter jug or have a filter tap installed at home. There's no definitive answer to how much water we should drink, but after a lot of reading and research I've come to the conclusion that two litres is about right.

☐ Start your day with water and keep a glass accessible at night.

☐ The darker your coffee roast, the better. Compounds released in the roasting process might inhibit the amalgamation of tau and amyloid beta, toxic proteins that play a key role in neurodegenerative conditions such as Alzheimer's and Parkinson's disease.

☐ I love a cup of builder's tea, especially first thing, but green tea has the greatest health benefits.[18] I brew a pot of loose-leaf green tea in the afternoon and keep it topped up with water as the day goes on. When I'm in an office, I throw a teaspoon of leaves into a mug and top with hot water (not boiling – it makes the tea bitter). They sink to the bottom of the mug as they hydrate, so there is no need to carry round an infuser.

9 Eat slowly, until 80 per cent full

Hara hachi bu is the Japanese instruction to eat until 'eight parts full', meaning: don't stuff your face until you can't eat another morsel. This is widely practised on the Japanese Blue Zone island of Okinawa, home to some of the world's longest-lived people. It's a way of creating calorific restriction without feeling too deprived. (Read more about the Blue Zones on page 38.)

☐ It's hard to know when you're exactly 80 per cent full. Eating slowly allows our satiety response to kick in. It takes about 20 minutes for our brain to receive the message that the stomach is full.

☐ Set the oven timer for 20 minutes when you sit down to eat. Eat a smallish portion, then stay at the table until the timer pings. How do you feel? Full? If you're still hungry, eat a little more. Take time to tune into your satiety cues.

☐ Make eating sociable whenever you can. We eat more slowly when we're with others, taking time to chat and engage.

☐ If you're eating alone, eat mindfully, without the distractions of phone, computer or TV. Try not to eat breakfast and lunch 'al desko'; many offices have a break-out area where staff can eat – make use of it.

10 Olive oil

Olive oil is the liquid gold of the Mediterranean diet. A four-and-a-half-year clinical study of older adults at risk of heart disease found that those eating an olive-oil-rich Medi diet had 30 per cent fewer instances of heart attacks, stroke and memory loss, and also improved blood pressure and cholesterol levels. It also triggers autophagy, the spring-cleaning process that clears out senescent and damaged cells,[19] and activates sirtuins, as we read about in Week 1.

☐ Two to three tablespoons of olive oil a day is all you need to make a difference to your health.

☐ A drizzle of olive oil on vegetables helps the gut to absorb nutrients. The oil itself is good for gut health, too.

☐ Use regular olive oil for sautéing and roasting vegetables at temperatures up to 220°C/425°F (beyond that it starts to degrade, and beneficial fatty acids break down).[20] Use cold extra virgin for salad dressings and drizzling.

☐ Rubbing a drop of olive oil on fingernails and cuticles keeps them shiny and healthy looking!

Nutrition tips to boost your week

The 10 daily habits on the previous pages will transform your health now and in the future. When you introduce them into your life you'll start to feel better almost immediately: lighter – with more energy and better digestion. But eating to age well doesn't stop there. There are plenty more actions you can take to make you feel amazing.

Tick each one when you've worked it into your week.

Pick pulses

Legumes or pulses – peas, beans and lentils – are fibre-packed nutritional powerhouses. When I kept my fibre diary, I found it hard to hit my target without a daily portion of beans. Research credits these cheap and easy superfoods with everything from lowering cholesterol levels to aiding weight loss.

☐ Tinned beans can help you get a meal on the table in minutes. Keep a variety in the larder: black beans, butter beans, chickpeas, black-eyed beans, kidney beans. I always have a couple of tins of each type tucked away.

☐ Buy a bag of red lentils. A couple of handfuls add fibre and protein to a soup or curry but are barely noticeable.

☐ If your family are pulse averse, try going 50:50 kidney beans and beef in a chilli, or mince and red lentils in a Bolognese.

☐ Try roasting or sautéing your cooked beans. Drain and rinse a tin of butter beans or chickpeas, mix with spices, one tablespoon of olive oil and a little salt. Sauté in a frying pan or roast in a hot oven until lightly browned and crispy.

Understand how nutrients work together to boost brain health

No one ever got healthy by focusing on just one food. All the broccoli in the world won't make up for a diet that's deficient in other areas. Recent research has revealed how a variety of nutrients work together for better cognitive performance.[21] Omega-3 fats, lycopene, carotenoids plus vitamins B12 and D interact to boost brain health. Make sure you're eating the following:

☐ Flax seeds, chia seeds and hemp seeds for omega-3 fats. However, the best source of omega-3 is oily fish (see overleaf).

☐ Tomatoes (particularly cooked ones), watermelon and red peppers provide lycopene.

☐ Sweet potatoes, carrots and squashes: their orange colour comes from carotenoids.

☐ Vitamin B12. It's found in meat and dairy (vegans need to supplement) and many people over 50 are deficient, which has been linked to depression[22] and cognitive decline.[23] In the US, people in this age group are recommended to supplement 2.4mcg per day. (See page 72 for more about vitamin D.)

Eat three portions of oily fish a week

By oily (fatty) fish, I mean salmon, mackerel, herrings, sardines, anchovies and, to a lesser extent, tuna (it can be high in mercury, and omega-3 levels vary depending on the type of tuna fish). These fish provide omega-3 essential fatty acids, which our bodies can't make. One study tracking omega-3 fatty acid levels in the blood found that for every 1 per cent increment there was a 20 per cent decreased risk in all-cause mortality.[24] Recent studies have found that people given omega-3 supplements had a decreased risk of a heart attack[25] and lower inflammatory markers.[26]

Omega-3s are also critical for brain health. Our neurons are coated with a fatty substance called myelin, which forms an insulating sheath, allowing the brain to send messages faster and more efficiently. Without fatty acids, myelin declines, leading to neurodegenerative diseases such as Alzheimer's, multiple sclerosis and Parkinson's.

☐ Tinned sardines (the cheap ones with the bones in, for extra calcium) are the ultimate age-well food. Eat them on toast for a quick lunch, or whizz them into a pâté with butter and watercress.

☐ Get wild salmon if you can. It's more expensive but it has higher levels of omega-3 than farmed salmon. Look out for tinned wild salmon and try the quick tinned salmon recipe on page 257.

☐ Experiment with salmon roe (eggs). Look out for it frozen or in jars at the fishmonger's, or buy online. It's expensive (and not to everyone's taste) but it's packed with DHA, a particularly potent omega-3 fatty acid that is vital for brain health.

☐ Buy a mackerel. They're cheap, sustainable and delicious. Bake a whole, gutted one in the oven for 25–30 minutes at 180°C/350°F/Gas 4 and eat with wholemeal bread, lemon wedges and a salad.

If you don't eat fish . . .

Walnuts, edamame, flax, chia and hemp seeds provide ALA. This is an omega-3 fatty acid, important for digestion and energy production. Our bodies can convert small amounts of ALA into DHA and EPA omega-3 fatty acids, but not in the quantities that we need for brain and heart health. Try a marine algae supplement to ensure an adequate supply of these vital nutrients.

Supplement with vitamin D

Our bodies need vitamin D to survive: it helps to build bone mass, support muscle strength, protect our respiratory system and maintain cognitive function. This powerful hormone (it's not really a vitamin at all) is synthesised when sunlight hits our skin, but we spend so little time outside that we rarely see enough natural light for this to happen. Add to that our bleak northern winters when the sun's UV wavelength is insufficient to create vitamin D, and our propensity to slather ourselves in sunscreen as soon as a few rays do break through, and it's no surprise that Public Health England recommends a supplement of 10mcg from autumn until spring, and all year if we don't get much sun. Research linking vitamin D sufficiency with an improved immune response to the coronavirus means I'll be taking it all year round. Make sure it's D3, not D2.

☐ Eat mushrooms. We can't get enough vitamin D solely from diet but mushrooms are a good source (and they're delicious!).[27] They also provide niacin, which helps the body to convert food into energy. Niacin also lowers levels of 'bad' cholesterol and triglycerides, reduces oxidative stress and inflammation, and boosts brain function.

☐ Vitamin D3 works with vitamin K2 to help calcium to reach, and strengthen, our bones.[28] You'll find K2 in liver, meat, eggs and full-fat dairy products.

A little sweetness

Too much sugar sends the body on an insulin roller coaster, creating inflammation and leading to weight gain, glucose intolerance and diabetes. And it's in everything. Many processed foods, such as bread and pasta sauces, contain refined sugar, or other sweeteners, such as corn syrup or anything ending in -ose. Read the ingredients list before you buy, and cook from scratch when you can. But a little sweetness from time to time won't kill you.

☐ Fill a couple of pitted dates with nut butter for a high-energy afternoon snack. Dates, particularly the medjool variety, are beautifully sweet and packed with fibre.

☐ Avoid natural sweeteners such as agave and maple syrup: they're still heavily processed foods and have the same impact on the body as refined sugar. Having said that, I do like a bit of maple syrup – see the recipe on page 271 – and a little goes a long way.

☐ Retrain your palate by cutting down on sugar. I used to love cheap chocolate and shop-bought cakes – now they taste weirdly artificial.

☐ Eat the birthday cake, drink the sticky cocktail. Life really is too short to agonise over every spoonful of sugar.

Dark chocolate (yay!)

The good news is that pretty much every nutritional expert, and every brain-health guru, recommends a little dark chocolate.

It's one of the most antioxidant-rich foods on earth, linked to everything from better cognition to improved heart health, and lower blood pressure to stronger cell membranes.

☐ Don't ignore the word 'dark' here. You need to buy chocolate that's at least 70 per cent cocoa solids. I've given up my (previously) beloved Dairy Milk.

☐ Melt a square or two of very dark chocolate on top of porridge for an extremely indulgent breakfast.

☐ I try to avoid so-called 'superfoods', but I do keep raw cacao powder and cacao nibs in my age-well larder. Cacao is the raw cocoa bean, with all the health benefits and none of the extra sugar or fat. I sprinkle the nibs on my breakfast pots.

☐ Check out the fantastic dark chocolate recipes on the agewellproject.com blog.

Fat is our age-well friend

The low-fat diets of the 1980s and 1990s are far behind us. Fat is vital to ageing well, and for delivering nutrients to help our brains and bodies to thrive. Unsaturated fats from avocados, nuts and olive oil deliver a range of health benefits. And saturated fats aren't the pariahs they once were. Focus on quality, not exact quantities: a marbling of fat in a beautiful steak rather than highly processed deli meats, a sliver of homemade cake made with butter rather than industrial cookies, a drizzle of olive oil rather than deep-fried anything.

☐ Cook with oils with a high smoke point, such as olive oil, rice bran oil and coconut oil. If your oil gets too hot and starts to smoke, ditch it and start again. Smoke indicates that the oil has degraded and produced trans fats (linked to high levels of 'bad' cholesterol).

☐ Don't ditch salad dressing: the oil helps the body to absorb nutrients. Use extra-virgin olive oil, walnut oil or avocado oil rather than a seed oil such as sunflower.

☐ Use a little fat to add texture to meals: avocado slices, a sprinkling of nuts, a drizzle of olive oil, a swirl of cream, a pat of butter.

☐ Try coconut oil to cook pancakes and curries. It's high in saturated fat but confers other health benefits. Research is still ongoing, however.

Alcohol? Yes, you can (probably)!

I've lost count of the number of people who have asked me, 'Can I age well and still have a drink?' The answer, in most cases, is 'yes', but it does depend on what and how you drink. Red wine has long been linked to longevity. Recent research has found that red wine drinkers have more diverse gut microbiota, and are less likely to be overweight or have high levels of 'bad' cholesterol.[29] A compound found in red wine, resveratrol, has been linked to slower ageing and lower stress levels.[30]

☐ Refer back to your family and personal health histories when you evaluate your relationship with alcohol. Red wine has been found to be beneficial for heart health, but if you have a risk of breast cancer, booze is not your friend. It doesn't help menopause symptoms either. Talk to your doctor about the risk factors.

☐ Drink mindfully. Be conscious of what you're doing and sip, don't glug. Make drinking a glass of wine a sociable activity with friends and loved ones, rather than something you do alone in front of the telly.

☐ Stick to government guidelines of drinking fewer than 14 units a week and remember that units aren't the same as glasses. There are two units in a 175ml glass of 12 per cent wine (most wines have a higher ABV – alcohol by volume) and just six pints of regular beer account for the recommended weekly total.

☐ Try a bottle-fermented beer. Some European beers are double fermented, making them probiotic-rich and good for gut health. Look for brands like Westmalle Tripel, Hoegaarden and Echt Kriekenbier, but be aware that they can contain almost twice as much alcohol as regular bottled beer. I can't finish a small bottle!

It's all nuts

Nuts are a wonder-food, providing unsaturated fatty acids, fibre, minerals and vitamins. Walnuts are age-well megastars, packed with omega-3 fatty acids which reduce oxidative stress and fight inflammation. And it's fitting that they're shaped like tiny brains – they boost brain health and may stimulate the development of new neurons. Our gut microbiota ferment the fibre in walnuts to create a short-chain fatty acid called butyrate, which has been linked to improved gut health, better sleep and reduced inflammation.

☐ A handful of nuts, about 30g, is the amount researchers recommend. A recent study linked eating this amount twice a week to a 17 per cent lower risk of death from heart disease.[31]

☐ Toasted nuts add a delicious crunch, and extra nutrients, to salads and vegetables dishes. When I'm prepping food, I'll often dry-roast some nuts in the oven (at 180°C/350°F/Gas 4 and for no more than 10 minutes – watch them like a hawk, or they'll burn) or toast them in a frying pan. The general rule is to toast round and crinkly nuts (hazelnuts, walnuts and so on) in the oven; flat seeds and chopped nuts (pumpkin seeds, flaked almonds) in a pan.

☐ Pesto isn't just for pine nuts. Whizz toasted walnuts, almonds or pumpkin seeds with herbs, garlic, lemon and olive oil to ring the changes.

☐ Check out agewellproject.com for Annabel's walnut-packed sticky toffee-pudding cake – it's so delicious and probably my family's favourite recipe on the whole site.

Don't ditch dairy

The subject of dairy comes up again and again when I'm giving workshops and coaching. Some people think it's the food of the devil and will give them cancer, whereas others feel that it's a wonder-food and they need huge portions each day. Neither is correct. Dairy has age-well benefits, but we don't need a lot of it. A small pot (150g) of plain live yogurt provides up to 30 per cent of our RDA of calcium, as well as probiotics, but there are other good sources of bone-building calcium out there: sardines with bones in (again), tofu, sesame seeds/tahini, beans and lentils.

☐ Add live natural yogurt to your diet. It's a good source of calcium, protein and gut-friendly probiota.

☐ Try kefir (fermented milk). It's a delicious addition to a breakfast bowl, or drink a small glass in the morning. It's also packed with probiotics.

☐ Enjoy a small portion of good-quality cheese, about 40g (a thumb-sized piece), particularly one of those made from raw milk (if your immune system can take it). They're anti-inflammatory, high in probiotics and contain spermidine, a compound which facilitates auto-phagy in the body.

☐ Avoid large quantities of processed cheese. It's high in salt and low in nutritional value.

How to make it work – pantry list

Here's a basic list of the items I keep in my kitchen to help me knock up age-well meals and snacks. You can find my complete pantry list in Appendix II if you want to stock up with everything I keep at home.

Larder

A wide variety of nuts, seeds and dried fruit, but always Brazil nuts, a fantastic source of selenium, which may quell inflammation caused by viruses.

Nut butters
Brown rice
Chia seeds
Dark chocolate (at least 70 per cent cocoa solids)
Flours: whole wheat, spelt, chickpea, buckwheat
Lentils and beans

Maple syrup
Oats – jumbo and porridge
Passata and tinned tomatoes
Quinoa
Tins of sardines and tuna
Wholewheat pasta, couscous and noodles

Avocados
Bananas, apples and seasonal fruit

Lemons and limes
Onions and garlic
Sweet potatoes and carrots

Black, green and herbal teas
Coffee

Herbs and spices, particularly
oregano, za'atar, baharat,
cinnamon, cloves, cumin,
sweet smoked paprika, and
turmeric

Apple cider vinegar
Coconut oil (raw, extra virgin)
Extra-virgin olive oil

Fridge

Anchovies
Eggs
Feta cheese
Ginger
Ground flax seeds
Hummus
Kefir
Plain live yogurt

Seasonal brassicas – broccoli,
sprouts, kale, cauliflower
Seasonal leafy greens – baby
spinach, cavolo nero
Soft herbs – coriander, basil,
flat-leaf parsley, mint
Tahini

Freezer

Blueberries
Chicken livers
Chopped spinach

Edamame beans
Tempeh
Wild salmon fillets

Miscellaneous

Beeswax wraps (to reduce waste and the amount of plastic that
comes into contact with food)
Water filter

The fibre content of top age-well foods

Food	Fibre content (g)	Quantity (typical portion size)
Baked beans in tomato sauce	7.4	200g
Kidney beans	6.6	120g
Chia seeds	5.7	1 tbsp (15g)
Chickpeas	5.5	120g
Porridge oats	5	50g
Jumbo oats	5	50g
Cannellini beans	4.5	80g
Soya beans (edamame)	4.2	80g
Banana	4.2	1 medium
Wholewheat spaghetti (cooked)	3.9	100g
Pear	3.7	1 medium
Multigrain bread	3.3	1 slice
Raspberries	3.2	50g
Kale	3.1	100g
Frozen peas	3	90g
Apple	2.9	1 medium
Seeded wholemeal bread	2.8	1 slice
Broccoli	2.3	100g
Spinach	1.8	80g
Mushrooms	1.2	100g
Brown rice (dry weight)	1.6	75g
Carrots (raw)	1.6	1 medium
Cauliflower	1.3	80g

Food	Fibre content (g)	Quantity (typical portion size)
Almonds, Brazil nuts	1.1	20g
Leek	1.1	1, white part only
Blueberries	0.8	50g
Cherries	0.8	50g
Strawberries	0.7	50g
Walnuts	0.7	20g

Your fibre diary/fibre tracker

Day	Food	Fibre content	Total
Sample day	Age-well breakfast bowl with oats, blueberries, nut butter and chia	10g	
	Lentil, spinach and butternut soup, slice of seeded brown bread	7g	
	Apple	2.9g	
	2 dates with 1 tbsp peanut butter	2.6g	
	Salmon, brown rice and green vegetables	6g	28.5g
Monday			

Day	Food	Fibre content	Total
Tuesday			
Wednesday			
Thursday			
Friday			

Day	Food	Fibre content	Total
Saturday			
Sunday			

Your age-well weekly menu planner

Below you will find my suggested menus for one week. You will find all the recipes, plus more information, in Appendix III starting on page 243.

Sunday
    Brunch: The Age-Well Fry-Up
    Dinner: Roast Chicken

Monday
    Breakfast: Classic Breakfast Pot
    Lunch: Sardines on Toast
    Dinner: Leftover Chicken Pho

Tuesday

    Breakfast: Black Forest Gateau Pot

    Lunch: Beans and Greens on Toast

    Dinner: Black Bean Chilli and Sweet Potato Tacos

Wednesday

    Breakfast: Sweet Green Smoothie

    Lunch: Brain-Boosting Salmon Salad with Kefir and Horseradish Dressing

    Dinner: Tempeh and Miso Stir-Fry

Thursday

    Breakfast: Spiced Tahini Granola

    Lunch: Chicken Liver and Pomegranate Salad

    Dinner: Thai Green Smoothie Curry

Friday

    Breakfast: Savoury Green Smoothie

    Lunch: Lentil, Feta and Chickpea Salad with Quick Pickled Red Onion

    Dinner: Green Dhal

Saturday

    Breakfast: Vegetable and Turmeric Muffins

    Lunch: Roast Squash and Pepper Soup with Ras-el-Hanout and Halloumi Croutons

    Dinner: Spiced Salmon with Pomegranate Molasses

Your personal age-well plan – diet

Review what you have achieved this week. How have you changed your diet? What's worked? What hasn't? What's been hardest? What's been easiest? What have you been eating? Which recipes have worked best for you?

I've listed the key actions again here to remind you. Tick the strategies that have worked well for you. There's a line for notes and reminders, too.

☐   Reduce ultra-processed food

☐   Cook at home

☐   Overnight fast

☐   Mediterranean diet – vegetables, pulses, whole grains

☐   Gut-healthy foods

☐   Work towards the recommended daily fibre target

☐   Eat more leafy greens

☐   Eat until 80 per cent full

☐   Focus on quality carbohydrates

☐   Three portions of oily fish per week

☐   Make olive oil your fat of choice

☐   Enjoy dark chocolate

Set your intentions for the future – diet

Based on the tick list you've just created, write out your dietary intentions. This will help you to stick to your age-well plan and create a list of good habits that will last you a lifetime; for example, *Every day I will eat one portion of berries, two portions of leafy greens and two tablespoons of olive oil*. This is your commitment to eat well to age well.

Look back to your personalised health plan from last week. How have you been able to act on your health plan this week? Write out your *purpose* again here to help you remember it:

DR LORI SHEMEK, AUTHOR AND DIET AND NUTRITION EXPERT

'Use intermittent fasting to age well'

Dr Lori Shemek is the Huffington Post's 'top diet and nutrition' expert, and the best-selling author of *How to Fight FATflammation!* Her latest book, *The Beginners' Guide to Intermittent Fasting*, is available on Kindle.

Lori's work on the role of inflammation in weight gain and ageing led her to focus on intermittent fasting (IF). She sees it as a natural progression: 'Research shows that intermittent fasting has the ability to help reverse and protect against inflammation. Chronic inflammation is the core underlying cause of most illness, disease, faster ageing and weight gain. Many people have excess inflammation because they are over-eating, and an excess of food creates inflammatory pathways.'

Like me, Lori believes that IF is a powerful age-well tool. It triggers autophagy, the essential cellular housekeeping that breaks down and recycles damaged molecules and cellular organelles. 'Purposeful intermittent fasting can reset our cells to a more youthful state', she explains. 'Many of the anti-ageing effects of IF come from autophagy. There are a number of mechanisms involved that reduce inflammation and oxidative stress.'

I asked her to clarify just how long she thinks a fast should be, because there is so much conflicting advice out there. 'The sweet spot of intermittent fasting occurs at 18 hours and beyond, as this is when we see the greatest drop in insulin and breakdown of fat. Longer fasts are of greater benefit but not practical for many; however, 12 hours of IF will provide great benefit as well.'

She advises people who are finding IF tough to focus on what's happening in their bodies. 'The body's always on a circadian rhythm, so if you eat breakfast every day at 9am, your stomach will growl at 9am. Once you understand that, no, you won't die because you're not eating, you will see and feel the difference! The largest obstacle is our mental barrier about not eating. If you know you're optimising health when you don't eat, then that helps to move you through the initial stage of fasting. You'll survive just fine without food.'

Lori's advice is to take it slowly when you start fasting: 'It's important to ease into it and allow your body to get used to not eating. Initially, prepare for intermittent fasting by reducing snacks until you are not snacking at all. The next step would be to delay breakfast (for example) by one hour every three or four days until you attain your fasting window goal.'

Her own fasting window varies depending on the day: 'I personally fast for 12–14 hours daily and 16 hours on the weekends.' Fasting isn't a substitute for healthy eating, though: 'It's very important to break your fast with good fats and protein such as nuts, avocado, whole eggs, or salmon to balance blood sugar.' Going from a fasted state to a huge meal of sugar and refined carbs would undo some of the benefits of fasting, and promote inflammation in the body, she explains.

Lori is evangelical about the importance of IF as we strive to age well. 'When we don't eat, the magic happens,' she says. 'It's one of the best tools we have to age well, and it's free!'

You can read more on drlorishemek.com

WEEK 3

How to Move

You've nailed eating well; now it's time to build on that foundation. This week you'll continue your age-well eating plan and add another layer, movement. There's no way round it: if we want healthy longevity, we have to find a way to fit movement into every waking hour of every day. And that means everything from fidgeting to pumping iron.

Keep moving, every hour, every day

We are not designed to live sedentary lives – and they're killing us. According to the WHO, sedentary behaviour now ranks among the top 10 leading causes of death. The average adult spends between 9 and 12 hours a day sitting.

Remember those nine 'hallmarks of ageing' from Week 1? We can mitigate all of them with exercise. And whatever it is you dread most about ageing – cardiovascular disease, cognitive decline, cancer, metabolic syndrome (the precursor to diabetes), frailty – the risk is reduced by movement. Physical fitness also boosts the fitness of our immune system to deal with viruses and pathogens, mobilising our white blood cells to seek and destroy. Most importantly, the more we exercise, the more likely we are to retain functional independence, and be able to look after ourselves, at any age.

As we exercise, our longevity genes shift our cells into survival mode. We're stressing our bodies (in a good way), so they wake up and get going, kick-starting our longevity pathways and activating sirtuins (refer back to page 25 if you need to remind yourself about these). These in turn protect our telomeres, help-ing them to grow.[1] Regular exercisers have longer telomeres, and this relationship is particularly clear as we get older, suggesting that physical activity has a role in combating the typical short-ening of telomeres which comes with age.[2]

Recent research by Cambridge University found that high levels of exercise resulted in a lower risk of death. The study revealed that taking up exercise after years of inactivity was a huge benefit to longevity. But the greatest age-well benefits were for those people who were doing plenty of exercise at the start of the study and increased it over time.[3] Wherever you're starting from – couch potato to marathon runner – there are ways to focus your routine for enhanced longevity.

This week we'll start by moving every hour of every day. We'll focus on the best exercise of all: walking; we'll wake up our mitochondria (the batteries of our cells) by getting a bit breathless, we'll fight frailty by building muscle, we'll stretch out and – trust me on this – we'll make it fun.

Before I committed to ageing well, working out was a long way down my to-do list, but everything I've learnt about healthy longevity and exercise has motivated me to get moving. This week you'll get motivated too, diarising exercise before anything else and sticking to your age-well goals.

Assess yourself as you start the week

The questionnaire below will give you an indication of your starting point. As with last week, there's no judgement, this is just an opportunity to evaluate. The fact that you're starting is important – this is where ageing well begins.

Questionnaire: how much are you moving now?

1 How many steps do you walk each week?

2 How many times do you get breathless each week? And for how long?

3 For how many hours do you sit down each day?

4 Where are you most sedentary? At work, watching TV in the evenings or on your commute, for example?

5 How much time do you spend outdoors? And how much of that time is in nature rather than on urban streets?

6 When did you last dance like nobody's watching?

7 How do you feel about your body? Fit or flabby?

8 How much exercise equipment do you have in your home? How often do you use it?

9 How often do you exercise with friends or family?

10 How often do you stretch?

By the end of this week you will:

- Understand the value of moving every hour.
- Be fidgeting and stretching all day, every day.
- Be walking with purpose, and faster.
- Get breathless and push yourself.
- Have started building more muscle.
- Make exercise fun – and learn to schedule it.
- Get outside more.
- Learn to love cold showers – honestly!

The big picture: movement – 5 essential lessons

Whatever your starting point, be gentle with yourself as you start to move to age well. I encourage you to get sweaty and breathless, but you must work to your own level. Consult your doctor if you're radically overhauling how much you move, deal with any injuries with the help of a professional and build up gradually.

1 Don't sit still for more than an hour

People in the Blue Zones move naturally throughout the day. Their environment, where they tend gardens, walk everywhere and go without the automated domestic appliances we rely on, nudges them to move every 20 minutes or so. Our environments keep us static, locked into chairs, at desks, slumped in front of a computer or lounging on a sofa in front of the TV.

Even when we do move, it's often in furious bouts at either end of the day, bookending long hours of stillness. Get up now and have a little walk around, stretch a bit, then come back to the book. It feels good doesn't it?

Recent research found that almost any level of activity – gentle walking, washing dishes, cooking – results in a lower risk of death.[4] And replacing just half an hour of sitting each day with that kind of low-intensity activity is linked to a 24 per cent reduced risk of death from cardiovascular disease.[5]

Sitting impacts every cell in our bodies. A study found that women who exercised for fewer than 40 minutes and were sedentary for more than 10 hours a day had biologically older cells than women who moved and exercised more. Specifically, the sedentary women had shorter telomeres than the more active ones.[6] Inactive women also have a greater cancer risk: the American Cancer Society found that women who sat for six or more hours a day had a 10 per cent higher risk of any cancer than those who sat for just three hours a day.

Think about those Blue Zoners we met in Week 1, moving every 20 minutes, and our own forebears who turned mangles, chopped wood and baked bread. Thank goodness we don't have to do all that any more, but our movement levels have plummeted as a result. We can, however, walk around the office, have a stretch or run an errand every hour.

2 How far can you walk each day?

Walking is the exercise equivalent of eating more vegetables: a baseline, non-negotiable, do-or-die activity (literally) to increase your chances of healthy longevity. Walking for two and a half hours a week (compared to no physical activity at all) reduces the risk of death from all causes by 20 per cent.

Ten thousand steps has become the gold standard for the amount of walking we should aim for each day. That's the quantity recommended by the WHO. But it's a totally arbitrary (although easily remembered) number, based on a 1960s marketing campaign in Japan for a prototype pedometer. Scientists disagree about the exact number we should aim for, but below 5,000 steps a day can lead to weight gain, loss of bone mass and muscle atrophy. At between 7,000 and 8,000 steps a day the health benefits start to kick in,[7] reducing the risk of cardiovascular disease, stroke and some forms of cancer.

A recent study of a group of adults with an average age of 73 found that 8,900 steps was the magic number to slow the rate of cognitive decline.[8] This level of exercise also slowed the rate of brain tissue loss among those members of the group who had high levels of amyloid plaque (a protein linked to Alzheimer's disease) in their brains.

The best and most obvious benefit of walking is that it's so easy and so readily accessible. We can all pull on a pair of comfortable shoes and walk. And then walk a little more. Daytime walking also gifts us the benefit of daylight, boosting vitamin D, sleep and mood. Think about each journey you make this week; could all – or part – of it include a walk? Can you extend a walk you already make, adding more steps to your day?

England's former Chief Medical Officer, Dame Sally Davies, advised, 'We need more active travel, we need people to get off the bus or the tube a stop early. We need people to climb stairs instead of getting in a lift … We need to be more active.' She added that there is 'no such thing as too little exercise', meaning that every little bit counts.

My age-well mantra

'Can I walk there?' I always ask myself this question when I'm running errands, dashing to an event after work or travelling between meetings. Often, I can walk the whole way (or at least part of it).

3 The power of breathlessness and HIIT

You don't need to be a marathon runner to reap the age-well benefits of exercise. All you need is to get a bit breathless. This means that whatever your current fitness level, you make gains when you push yourself a little harder. Just as being hungry puts the body under stress, so does being breathless. It's that level of challenge that activates longevity genes and boosts mitochondrial activity. Pushing yourself to breathlessness also increases

BDNF (brain-derived neurotrophic factor), which acts like fertiliser for your brain.

Vigorous exercise has also been found to increase the grey matter in the brain.[9] The volume of our grey matter mirrors our ability to do certain types of brainwork, including focusing and recalling. A decline in grey matter is associated with dementia and cognitive decline.

The good news is that this intensive activity doesn't need to be sustained for long. Working out to get breathless, and then taking a break to recover, is often referred to as HIIT: high-intensity interval training. It sounds intense – the clue's in the name – but it's easy to do, whatever your fitness level.

How to HIIT

HIIT can be fitted into almost any exercise plan. If you like cycling, running, swimming, walking, going to the gym or working out at home, you can HIIT as you go.

HIIT simply means short bursts of intense activity followed by a more leisurely pace. And what constitutes vigorous activity for one person is – literally – a walk in the park for another.

What to do Aim for 10–20 minutes three times a week. Go at your usual pace for a couple of minutes, then add a burst of speed and intensity for 10–20 seconds, then back to your usual pace for two minutes, then speed up again. Repeat this pattern for 10 minutes and try to build up to 20.

4 Muscle v. frailty – weights and resistance training

After the grand old age of 30, we typically start to lose muscle mass. This is a natural process associated with ageing, and it happens to everyone, usually at a rate of between 3 and 8 per cent a year. After the age of 50, the process accelerates, so muscle mass can decline between 30 and 50 per cent between 40 and 80 years of age. Severe muscle loss is known as sarcopenia and is a key factor in the frailty, falls and fractures we associate with old age. Building strength and endurance are our best defence by slowing bone loss and muscle wastage.

We need to work our muscles and keep strengthening them to counteract this natural decline. There's no easy way round it: as our muscles waste, we have to build them back up again if we want to age well. And everything we do to work our muscles, works our bones too. Like our muscles, they decline as we age, responding to activity or inactivity. Each time we move, our bones react to gravity and muscle contraction, rebuilding and remodelling themselves. If we're not moving, they're not strengthening.

Strength training helps to improve sleep quality, reduces the risk of heart attacks, strokes and type-2 diabetes, and eases the pain of arthritis. One study found that older adults who did strength training at least twice a week had almost 50 per cent lower odds of death from all causes, compared with those who did no strength training. They also had a 41 per cent lower risk of cardiac death and a 19 per cent lower risk of dying from cancer.

Resistance training refers to any form of exercise that builds muscle endurance. The resistance comes from your own body weight – a push-up or squat, for example – from free weights such as dumbbells, or from machines in the gym. Weight training involves lifting a weight to build strength. Both have unique health and fitness benefits that can't be gained from any other type of exercise. Swimming and other ways of working out in water, such as aquarobics, are also forms of resistance training.

If you haven't done it before, strength training might sound scary. I was rather terrified when I first stepped into the gym to work with weights. I still feel a bit silly, to be honest, and out of place among the sweaty lads in singlets. But I asked an instructor to show me how to use the machines and I worked out a routine based on my capabilities. And now I like having biceps!

5 Yoga, Pilates and stretching

Yoga developed over 5,000 years ago as a way to prepare the mind and body for meditation. More recently, it's evolved with a focus on exercise, strength, flexibility and breathing.

A review of 22 studies into the impact of yoga on longevity found that, for people over 60, practising yoga helped to improve balance, flexibility and limb strength. It also reduced depression, improved sleep quality and boosted vitality.[10]

Research published at the end of 2019 linked the practice to increased brain health. A review of 11 studies found that yoga might keep the brain healthy, boost memory and lower the risk of neurodegenerative diseases such as Alzheimer's. The researchers reported an increase in the size of the hippocampus, which is linked to memory, in regular yoga practitioners, as well as beneficial brain changes in the amygdala, which regulates emotions and boosts happiness. As we age, these two brain regions shrink, eventually leading to cognitive decline.

It's not clear exactly how yoga benefits the brain. But it might be linked to the reduction in stress that comes from regular practice. People who did yoga for eight weeks had a lower cortisol response to stress, and performed better on decision-making and attention tests.

The most important thing to remember is it's having a go that counts. I'm not sure where I read this great quote, but it encapsulates the idea that we should just give the practice a try: 'Saying you're not flexible enough to do yoga is like saying you're too dirty to have a bath.' Think about it!

If yoga isn't your thing, or it's too hardcore for your current state of fitness, consider Pilates or other ways to work stretches into your routine. Pilates focuses on strength and stability and may work better for you if you're recovering from injury. However you do it, keeping mobile and flexible is critical as we get older, reducing the stiffness that often comes with ageing.

How I make it work – making exercise fun

Five years ago, I was approaching 50, unfit and flabby. I wasn't a particularly sporty kid and exercise hadn't become part of my life as I got older. But learning about the impact of exercise on longevity and working out my purpose, have made a huge difference. Those two things get me out of bed to go for a jog or to the gym. I'm not running marathons, but I do have some biceps I'm proud of, and I feel fitter than ever.

I've learnt to make exercise a part of my life by taking ownership of it. And not to be put off when I'm the oldest in the class, or when the class is full of skinny yummy-mummies in the latest gear. (Having said that, if you want to splash out, having a few nice bits of exercise wear is very motivational!)

I schedule a week ahead, so I know I can fit my week around my workouts. And, most importantly, I make sure it's not all sweating in the gym and running in the rain. I make it fun!

- Go dancing with friends on a Friday night (explain to them that it doesn't matter how bad you all are – see page 113 for why).
- Play ping-pong with teenagers (see page 113 for the benefits).
- Never go for a *coffee* with a friend – go for a *walk* with a friend. You can pick up a coffee on the way.
- Smile and chat to people in the gym. If you go to the same class regularly, you'll get to know people. We've noticed that the twenty-somethings don't make it to the early gym classes on weekend mornings, so the over-forties have them to themselves! It's very social.
- Get your partner involved. I know this can be tough, but having the goal of ageing well together is the greatest gift you can give your relationship. If your other half is resistant, explain to them how important ageing well is to you, and your sense of purpose.

The Top 10: move to age well every day

Introducing a little more movement into every day will change the way you age. Below are ten small, but mighty, actions that won't eat into your schedule. Some only take seconds, most you can do while you're doing something else, and all of them will make a huge difference to your body. Set some reminders, and get started. Tick off each one you achieve and write down any concerns, notes and ideas underneath each section.

1 The muscle you might have forgotten

When did you last give your pelvic floor a workout? It's a complex mesh of muscles (imagine a 3-D hammock and you'll get the idea), supporting the pelvis and spine. It controls both the bladder and the bowel, and assists with sexual satisfaction for both men and women. Fifty per cent of post-menopausal women, and 25 per cent of men over 50, suffer urinary incontinence,[11] but it's rarely discussed as a health issue as we age. I talked to Myra Robson, the physio behind the app Squeezy, which teaches pelvic exercises and reminds us to do them. Myra explained that it might be *common* to leak as we get older, but it's not *inevitable*. Exercises can make a huge difference. These are Myra's tips for a daily pelvic workout:

- For women, start by squeezing the muscles around your back passage, then tighten around the vagina and urethra (where you pee from) as if you're trying to stop yourself from passing urine. It should feel like a squeeze and lift inside. After each squeeze and lift make sure you fully relax the muscles before you start again.
- For men, Myra advises thinking 'nuts to guts' or 'testicles to spectacles' to get the squeeze right!

☐   A pelvic-floor workout should be a mixture of long, slow holds and short, pulsing squeezes. The standard programme consists of 10 slow squeezes lasting 10 seconds each with a four-second rest between each one; and 10 fast squeezes at a speed of one per second.

The key is to do it regularly: six times a day if you have continence issues, three times a day as a preventative measure. Use the Squeezy app or set a reminder elsewhere so you don't forget.

Myra warns that it's always easy to do the quick squeezes, but it's the slow long holds that really make a difference. Give your pelvic floor the focus it deserves.

2 Fidget

We grew up being told not to fidget, but as adults it's one of the best things we can do for our health! It's a simple way to counteract the sedentary nature of our day. Research into the movements of over 12,000 women found that the fidgeters lived longer. The correlation was strong enough to cancel out the increased mortality associated with sitting for long periods.[12]

☐   Embrace your inner wriggly child, and fidget while you're sitting today. There's no wrong way to do it, just have a wriggle and a bit of a stretch.

☐   Fidget every hour, on the hour.

☐   If you want to go further, try the desk-side workout below.

3 Stretch: my desk-side workout

Sitting at a desk for hours at a time is one of the worst things we can do for our health, but work and other responsibilities keep us there. Use the time to get moving.

- [ ] When you are able to take a moment between tasks, stretch and move.

- [ ] Stand up for phone calls and to talk to colleagues who come to your desk.

- [ ] Walk around the office as much as you can, and make use of break-out spaces to eat and do specific pieces of work.

- [ ] Try this workout at your desk, either sitting or standing:

  - Start at the top of your head, moving it from side to side and up and down to loosen out your neck muscles.
  - Roll your shoulders backwards and forwards. Stretch your arms out to the side and up to the ceiling, circling your wrists as you do so.
  - Point one arm down to the floor and the other up to the ceiling, tilt in the direction of the arm pointing downwards so that you feel a stretch in your obliques (the side of your waist). Repeat on the other side.
  - Put your arms down and wiggle your hips from side to side.
  - Clench and relax your buttocks three times.
  - Lift each leg, straighten it out and rotate your foot.

Put your feet on the ground and roll through each one, from toe to base of heel and back again. Workout completed!

4 Make your walking brisk

It's not enough to stroll through your daily walk. To help us age well, walking must be brisk and purposeful. Research analysing the walking speeds of over 50,000 people in the UK and correlating them with mortality rates found that participants aged 60 or over more than halved their risk of death from cardiovascular diseases if they walked fast.[13]

☐   Fast walking can be any pace that gets you a bit sweaty and out of breath after a while.

☐   Walk every day, the more steps the better.

5 Build a 'home gym'

Can you dedicate a small area of your home to exercise? I'm not talking about a state-of-the-art home gym here, but a corner where you know you can move and stretch, and there's space to stash some basic equipment. You really don't need much: a simple in-house starter kit (kept all in one place) will help to establish your intentions and keep you consistent.

This means it's close at hand when you have a spare five minutes to exercise. And that's all it takes to make a difference. A few ideas for your workout starter kit:

☐   A yoga mat

☐   A pair of hand weights – 1.5kg (3lb 5oz) or 2kg (4½lb) is a good place to start. Mine are 2kg (4½lb); my husband's are 3kg (6½lb).

☐   Kettlebells – sets are cheap online, or just buy one. Mine is 8kg (17½lb).

☐   Resistance bands in different strengths.

6 Rethink your commute

Whether you're commuting to work or running errands, working movement into this dead time can be hugely beneficial. I stopped taking the bus to the tube and now cycle to the station instead. I make sure that I get some steps in before I get to work too, getting off the tube a stop early so that I can walk (briskly) to my desk.

☐   Think about each of the journeys you make in a day. How can you work more movement into all of them?

☐   If you're on a bus or train, work some of the desk-side workout above into your journey. Everyone else is glued to their screens, so they won't notice you wriggling around!

☐   Bought groceries? Use the bags for a weighted workout by doing biceps curls.

☐ Haven't got a seat? Hold on to a handrail and do calf raises, rising up onto your toes and then lowering again. Engage your core muscles to keep you stable.

☐ Have you got a seat? Imagine you need to flex every single muscle in your body. Begin by wiggling your toes and then contract and relax each muscle, one at a time, for three seconds, until you reach the top of your head.

7 Embrace cold showers

Don't hate me, but – as with fasting and intense exercise – bursts of cold put our longevity pathways under the right kind of stress. The pathways send signals to our cells to start repairing – exactly what we want to happen as we age. Getting cold activates our mitochondria and supports our immune system. A Dutch study of 3,000 people found that those who took cold showers every morning were 30 per cent less likely to take time off sick. When they added regular physical activity, sick days reduced by over 50 per cent.[14] A daily cold shower also lowers inflammation, stimulates the vagus nerve (see page 188) and resets the nervous system. I do it every day now and find it invigorating. If I skip a day, I miss it.

☐ Start slowly and talk to your doctor first if you have any health issues.

☐ Enjoy your warm shower, then turn the thermostat down for 30 seconds. Don't go all the way down first time – take it gradually.

☐ Thirty seconds is enough to make a difference, then turn the thermostat back up and get warm.

☐ If you're feeling hardcore, do it again!

8 Make brushing your teeth a brain and body workout

Cleaning our teeth is such a basic part of our personal-hygiene routine that we tend to forget its age-well benefits. Multiple studies link gum disease to dementia: bacteria associated with chronic gum disease are found in the Alzheimer's brain. Those bacteria secrete a toxic protein, gingipain, which seems to destroy neurons.[15] Brush your teeth well for better brain health!

Use the time spent brushing your teeth for a mini workout:

☐ If your balance is good enough, stand on one leg as you brush your teeth. It strengthens the ankles and improves balance. Make sure there's something to hold on to in case you wobble! My electric toothbrush runs in 30-second bursts for two minutes, so I switch legs each time.

☐ Use your non-dominant hand to hold your toothbrush. It activates the parts of the brain used in learning and memory.

☐ Don't forget to floss afterwards: many gerontologists list flossing as one of their top tips for healthy ageing. It helps to prevent the build-up of the bacteria that cause gum disease.

9 Jump for your bones!

After the age of 40 we lose bone mass at the rate of 1 per cent a year. That doesn't sound a lot, but by 60 it's starting to add up. Exercise doesn't just build muscle – it builds bone, too. Our bones constantly rebuild and remodel themselves, adapting to whatever comes their way – whether that be activity or inactivity. Research indicates that jumping may be the best exercise to build strong bones, but please don't try it if you are suffering from osteopenia or osteoporosis, or if you have issues with your balance or joints/ligaments. Try these ways to build bone strength:

☐ Try to jump between 10 and 20 times a day. I jump around while I'm getting dressed and have worked star jumps and burpees into my six-minute workout – see page 111.

☐ Running and resistance training also build strong bones.

☐ If this all sounds too hardcore, or your bones and joints aren't up to it, try trampolining, t'ai chi or dancing, all of which improve postural control.

☐ Swimming isn't a weight-bearing exercise, but it leads to higher bone turnover, and thus stronger bones. Swimming is a great way to boost cardiovascular fitness and muscle strength without impact stress on the body.

10 Create a six-minute workout

Few of us have time to do a full workout every day (and if you do, make sure you schedule rest days). But six minutes? That's easier to find. I urge you to carve out six minutes from your day and use it to move. It's important to do something that works for you, at your fitness level, without the risk of injury. Make sure you're wearing comfy clothes and supportive trainers. And set a timer to keep you on track. Try these:

☐ Pick two of your favourite tracks and dance around to them. Have a break between the two if you need to.

☐ Use the time to do the desk-side stretching routine outlined on page 105.

☐ Use your hand weights or kettlebells to create a workout.

☐ I do a six-minute circuit combining cardio, core and conditioning. I warm up first and stretch afterwards so that makes it a bit longer.

My six-minute circuit

I get some music going and set a one-minute timer on my phone. I restart the timer as soon it as goes off and move straight on to the next exercise. I try to do different exercises each time, so I work a variety of muscles across the week.

It's important to do the following exercises properly to avoid injury and ensure that you get the full benefit. You will find many videos on YouTube with clear explanations. Here's a sample circuit:

- Minute 1 **cardio** – star jumps
- Minute 2 **conditioning** – push-ups
- Minute 3 **core** – sit-ups
- Minute 4 **cardio** – burpees
- Minute 5 **conditioning** – alternate-leg lunges
- Minute 6 **core** – plank

Don't do jumping exercises unless your knees and joints are up to it and don't forget to stretch and warm up and down!

Exercise tips to boost your week

You'll be moving more every day, but you still need to schedule time for longer workouts. Three weekly sessions of exercise of around 40–45 minutes each is a good target. Variety really is the spice of life when it comes to exercise: working a range of different types of movement into your week will reap huge age-well benefits. See page 119 for how I schedule my week to fit in more exercise and page 120 for a one-week movement diary that will enable you to do the same.

Tick each one when you've worked it into your week.

Dance – and why it's good to be bad

A review of all the sports and activities undertaken by 1,000 older Japanese women found that dancing was the only one to reduce the risk of functional decline (for example, being unable to wash or eat unaided). Researchers put this down to the unique combination of balance, strength, endurance, memory and concentration that dance requires.[16] Even better, you don't need to be good at dancing for it to be a brain workout: learning new steps builds new neurons, whereas repeating the same moves over and over has no benefits.

☐ Find a dance class near you and enrol. Just give it a go, and feel positive about the experience. However bad you perceive yourself to be, you're benefiting from it.

☐ Try a variety of different styles: salsa, samba, ballroom, ballet, tap – the more the better. Or try Zumba or other dance fitness classes that are good fun.

☐ If you can, dance with a variety of partners – it works the brain harder.

☐ Pick a few favourite tracks at home and dance like nobody's watching.

Ping-pong!

Table tennis is one of the best exercises to fend off dementia. The rapid movements, hand–eye coordination and complex thinking skills it requires make it a full brain–body workout. And it's always a laugh. We have a table in the garden. If you don't have space, seek out community tables – you might find some in your local park.

☐ Plan weekly table tennis.

Muscle bound?

England's Chief Medical Officer (CMO) recommends two sessions of strengthening exercises a week. Weight and resistance training increases metabolism, lowers body fat and reduces the risk of frailty and diabetes. Multiple studies have found that having good muscle strength in midlife is one of the best predictors of a longer lifespan. How are you going to fit in your two sessions a week?

☐ Your body is the best resistance machine you have: try lunges, squats and push-ups.

☐ Challenge your muscles to the point of exhaustion: it's the last repetition you can do without losing form that stimulates muscles to grow.

☐ Check out circuit classes at your local gym and talk to the instructor about your fitness level.

☐ You can break down these sessions into smaller bites: just a couple of minutes of exercising with the weights in your 'home gym' can make a difference if you do it regularly.

Time to stretch – yoga and Pilates

The benefits of yoga are spelt out on page 100. Whatever your starting point, yoga and Pilates have the power to strengthen the body and calm the mind. Go slowly to start with, talk to your instructor about your capabilities – and remember to breathe.

☐ Many yoga and Pilates studios have classes specifically for beginners or older people. See what's available in your area.

☐ If you can't get to a studio, look online for a class. I like Yoga with Adriene on YouTube and have a very simple free app on my phone called Sun Salutations.

☐ One class a week is a great start.

Take a walk on the wild side

Put aside some time this weekend for a long walk somewhere with a bit of greenery. Go by yourself for some deep-thinking time, listen to an informative podcast or take a friend (see below for the benefits of walking with a friend). It's terrific exercise, provides all the benefits of daylight and gets you out in nature (see page 210).

☐ Have you scheduled your long walk?

Make it social

All these exercises are more fun with friends, or in a class. There's something about group activity that pushes us a bit harder, and releases more post-workout endorphins.

☐ Try a group workout class, walking with friends or a sociable dance session this week.

Get sweaty 1: HIIT

However you do it, you need to get a sweat on this week. Three sessions of HIIT (page 98) is ideal, but one is a great start. There are so many benefits to aerobic activity: recent research showed that older adults at risk of Alzheimer's (due to family history or genetic predisposition) who ran on a treadmill three times a week for six months improved both cardio fitness and brain function.[17]

☐ Try the HIIT routine outlined on page 98 on the running or rowing machine at your gym.

☐ Work HIIT into a walk or jog.

☐ I try to HIIT while I'm on my bike (on empty roads), too.

☐ Have you found a six-minute workout (see page 111) that's working for you? Extend it to 12 minutes, 18 minutes, 24 minutes. Have a one-minute break between each session and drink plenty of water.

Get sweaty 2: sauna (or steam)

I'm not suggesting you go out and build a sauna in the garden (although people do), but if you have access to a sauna, at your gym or a local spa, give it a go. Large studies, particularly in Finland (where they like a sauna), show strong links between sauna use and a lower risk of age-related conditions, including cardiovascular disease and cognitive decline. In much the same way as intensive exercise, working up a sweat with steam or dry heat has been shown to repair cellular damage, which could otherwise lead to cardiovascular or neurodegenerative disease.

☐ Take a sauna or steam this week. Start with five minutes and build up from there if your health is up to it. You reap the greatest cardiovascular benefits after 20 minutes.[18] The hardy Finns alternate time in the sauna with rolling in the snow or ice baths.

Work out in a fasted state

Think you need to fuel up before exercise? Think again. A recent study revealed that overweight men who worked out *before* breakfast burnt double the calories of those who worked out *after* breakfast. Those who worked out in a fasted state for six weeks also had better blood sugar regulation, potentially lowering diabetes and heart disease risk.

☐ Exercise before you breakfast. Now you're eating breakfast later, you're spending more time in a fasted state, so there's more time to work out on an empty stomach.

Five tips for exercising safely

Take it slowly and don't go too far beyond your comfort zone; you've got the rest of your life to work out, remember. If adding more movement, cold showers, hot saunas or working out in a fasted state is a big step for you, talk to your GP first and get advice from fitness staff at a gym or yoga studio if you go down that route.

1 Stay hydrated. Working out requires plenty of water.

2 Don't work out through pain. If you think you're injured, rest and consult a doctor/physio.

3 Have at least one rest day to allow muscles to rest and repair. I usually take two a week.

4 Stretch before and after exercise – this is increasingly important as we get older.

5 Don't just do one type of exercise – complement cardio or high-impact workouts with more gentle, stretch-based movement such as yoga or Pilates.

How to make it work – exercise

Every day I try to do a six-minute workout, stretch, fidget, have a cold shower, walk for 30 minutes in daylight (I've made that part of my commute) and jump!

Apart from yoga, the classes I do are all early morning, so I'm working out on an empty stomach. This is my best possible week (sometimes life gets in the way)!

My exercise week

Day	Morning	Evening	Duration	Location
Monday	A gentle run with HIIT intervals		30–40 minutes	Outside in the park or by the river
Tuesday	Rest day			
Wednesday	Resistance and weights circuit class		45 minutes	Gym
Thursday	HIIT boxing class	Yoga	45 minutes / 1 hour	Gym / Yoga studio
Friday	Rest day	Dancing with friends or ping-pong in the garden in summer		
Saturday	Resistance and weights circuit class	Yoga	45 minutes / 1 hour	Gym / Yoga studio
Sunday	Long walk or gentle run		1 hour	Somewhere green

Your age-well week – exercise

Schedule your exercise for this week. You're more likely to stick to it if you've planned ahead.

Day	Morning	Evening	Duration	Location
Monday				
Tuesday				
Wednesday				
Thursday				
Friday				
Saturday				
Sunday				

Your personal age-well plan – exercise

Review what you've achieved this week. How have you worked more movement into each day? What's worked? What hasn't? What's been hardest? What's been easiest?

I've listed the key actions again here to remind you. Tick the strategies that have worked well for you. There's a space for notes and reminders, too.

☐   Get moving – fidgeting and stretching at your desk.

☐   A 30-minute walk in daylight.

☐   Dancing.

☐   A daily six-minute workout.

☐   High-intensity interval training – at your level.

☐   Yoga or stretching.

☐   Exercise with friends.

☐　Weights and/or resistance training.

☐　Pelvic floor exercise.

☐　Cold showers.

☐　Workout in a fasted state.

☐　Jumping or other bone-strengthening exercise.

Set your intentions for the future – exercise

Based on the tick list you've just created, write out how you're going to work exercise into your life. This will help you to stick to your planned workout. For example, *Every day I will do a six-minute workout, stretch at my desk and have a hot–cold–hot shower.* Set your intentions: they will help you to create a list of good age-well habits that will last a lifetime.

Refer back to your age-well goals, personalised health plan and age-well eating plan from the last two weeks. Have you been able to maintain eating to age well this week?

Write out your *purpose* again here to help you remember it:

EXPERT INTERVIEW

JANE BAKER, FOOT AND ANKLE SPECIALIST, PHYSIOTHERAPIST

'Help your feet to age well'

Jane Baker is one of Britain's leading foot and ankle specialist physios with over 30 years' experience and a Harley Street practice. Her message to us as we age is clear: 'meet your feet'. These incredibly complex structures, each comprising 22 bones, 33 joints and over 7,000 sensory nerve endings, languish a long way from our brains and are encased in shoes throughout our waking hours. We often neglect them.

We may not need our feet in the way that our ancestors did – to support us to carry water and forage for food – but Jane says our feet are the foundation of our physical health, particularly as we get older. 'If something is slightly out of alignment, it triggers a "butterfly effect", causing problems throughout the body,' she explains. Jane's own passion for foot health started when, as a more general physiotherapist, she realised that many of the problems her patients were experiencing elsewhere in their bodies were linked directly to their feet.

'Touch your feet every day,' she urges. 'Take a few moments to focus on your feet as you towel off after a bath or shower, massaging the muscles to wake them up and give them some attention.' She also suggests rolling a soft ball under the arch of each foot daily. 'It's a really good way to stimulate sensory nerve endings and muscles.'

Foot pain, bunions, corns and other issues aren't inevitable, despite being very common. We shouldn't put up with them as we age, but we should seek treatment and help from doctors, physios and podiatrists, Jane explains. Our footwear should be supportive, particularly if we suffer pain in our feet or have collapsed arches. Simple things, such as making sure our shoes are the right size and fit, and checking that the heels are not worn down on one side, can make a big difference.

At 53, Jane is a keen kite-surfer, triathlete and skier, and puts particular emphasis on exercising her feet before each event or trip. But we all need to focus on mobility, strength and balance in our feet and ankles, whatever our fitness levels. Jane demonstrates, with her own muscular feet, tanned from a recent kite-surfing trip to Kenya, simple mobility exercises for our toes. She flexes them back and forth, spreading, curling and lifting them off the ground. 'Can you pick up a sock with your toes?' she asks. She also suggests mobilising ankles regularly by pumping them back and forth, then circling them.

We need mobility and strength in our feet and ankles to

propel our bodies forward as we walk, and to support our body weight. 'Walking,' Jane explains, 'is a controlled series of coordinated movements. Think of actors on stage: if one of them gets the timing wrong, the whole performance is in trouble.' Walking and running are single-leg activities – we balance on one leg, and then the other, as we move forward – so if we can't balance well on one leg it will affect the whole walking process and lead to an increased risk of falls and frailty. 'Balance atrophies as we age and the nervous system becomes sluggish,' Jane explains. 'We need to safely challenge our balance on a daily basis.' Try standing on one leg to clean your teeth, throw and catch a ball and touch the ground. 'Don't get complacent!' she laughs.

Read more at janebakerphysio.com.

WEEK 4

How to Sleep

When we first started the Age-Well Project, I thought that if I ate nutritious food and maybe moved a bit more, I'd be well on the way to healthy longevity. The greatest revelation to me, however, has been the critical role that sleep plays in how we age. You've done incredible work overhauling your eating and exercise patterns, so continue those powerful changes as we move onto sleeping to age well.

Sleep saves us

I've had problems sleeping well for a couple of decades: I stumbled from the sleeplessness of early motherhood to the sleeplessness of perimenopause and the sheer frazzlement of being a 'sandwich woman', caught between young children and a dependent parent. Since my mother died, and now that my children are older, I've been able to focus on quality sleep. I've learnt to treat the pursuit of sleep like a job, or an expensive hobby – cricket or fly-fishing, for example – that requires a lot of kit and a lot of time.

It's widely believed that we need less sleep as we age: some people do, but some don't. What's clear is that quality sleep is critical as we age, regulating brain function, metabolism, hormones and the cardiovascular system. In turn, a lack of shut-eye is linked to all the chronic conditions of ageing. Sleep deprivation is a significant risk factor for type-2 diabetes (and this in turn leads to erratic sleep patterns, creating a vicious cycle),[1] Alzheimer's disease, stroke, depression, high blood pressure and obesity. Tiredness results in the production of more ghrelin, the hunger hormone. Research has found that people eat 300 extra calories, and twice as much fat, after a bad night.[2]

As we age, our circadian rhythms, the biological clock that defines our sleep patterns, becomes disrupted. They fall victim to the same faltering epigenetic signalling that impacts our DNA.[3] A second 'clock' develops, knocking the first out of kilter. This, in turn, disrupts production of melatonin – a hormone made in the pineal gland in response to cues from the circadian rhythms and light exposure that instructs our body to bed down for the night. With our clocks going haywire, and melatonin production out of whack, it's no surprise that the rate of cell senescence (the zombie cells described on page 23) rises, increasing the pace of ageing in our bodies.

It's not all doom and gloom, however. This week we'll focus on getting a good night's sleep, prioritising bedtime, creating the right environment for sleep and supercharging your day to make night-time better.

Assess yourself as you start the week

It's important to know what's normal for you when it comes to sleep. We all have different sleep requirements at different times in our lives. But most of us know when we've had enough sleep to face the day ahead: we feel rested and able to cope. And most of us will have problems at some stage in our lives: a third of the global population has sleep issues at one time or another. Review your current sleep quality in the context of what's normal for you.

Questionnaire: how are you sleeping now?

1   How did you feel when you woke up this morning? Rested or exhausted?

2   How many hours of sleep did you get?

3   How many hours of sleep have you averaged over the last week?

4   Do you sleep better or worse now than you did a year ago? Five years ago?

5   What time do you normally go to bed?

6 What time do you normally get up?

7 How much time do you spend staring at a screen in the evenings?

8 What's your wind-down routine?

9 Do you take any supplements or medication to help you sleep?

By the end of this week you will:

- Have a sleep routine that works for you.
- Understand what's happening in your brain as you sleep.
- Seek blue light in the morning, and avoid it before bedtime.
- Have a sleep environment that makes you feel good about going to bed.
- Know what foods help you sleep.
- Have created a wind-down routine that gets you ready for sleep.
- Be able to cope with night-time waking.
- Set an alarm at night – and in the morning.
- Calm anxiety around not sleeping.

The big picture: sleep – 5 essential lessons

It's a fallacy that when we go to sleep our bodies shut down. In fact, they're as busy as ever, healing and repairing while we're in the land of Nod. We might not be aware that it's happening, but the time we're asleep is vital to the processes that help us age well.

1 Understand what happens in your brain as you sleep

I've mentioned quality sleep, but what does that mean? For most adults in middle age and beyond, it means seven to eight hours sleep a night (not necessarily continuously – see page 149), but you know when you feel rested, and when you don't. We need a combination of REM (rapid eye movement) and non-REM sleep, also known as slow-wave sleep or SWS, to give our brains the rest they need. If there's one thing that has motivated me to focus on sleep it's understanding the processes that happen in my brain as I slumber, particularly in relation to Alzheimer's disease risk.

We cycle through all stages of SWS and REM sleep five times during a typical night, with each cycle lasting around 90 minutes on average (but, again, we're all different). Slow-wave sleep takes us from waking into deep sleep in three stages, and it's in deep sleep that we get the most effective rest, consolidating memories. We get more of this kind of sleep during the first part of the night. Increasingly longer, deeper periods of REM sleep occur towards morning. It's during REM sleep that we dream, with our brain in a highly active state that appears to be part of the process of creating memories and processing emotions.

As we sleep, our brains go into housekeeping mode, with their in-built cleaning team, the glymphatic system, clearing out toxins that accumulate during the day. Recent research shows that microglia – immune cells that act as brooms to sweep accumulated toxins out of the brain – work much more effectively while we sleep.[4] The sleeping brain is also better at removing the amyloid-beta protein that is implicated in Alzheimer's. As we enter deep sleep, the brain physically alters, with cells shrinking up to 60 per cent to allow cleaning between them – the neurological equivalent of shifting the furniture around when you give the house a spring clean!

It's unsurprising, therefore, that poor sleep quality has been linked to a build-up of the amyloid-beta plaques found in Alzheimer's disease. Research on people in their seventies found that those who reported sleeping less had elevated levels of amyloid beta. And when participants in a study were allowed to sleep, but disturbed enough to prevent them entering deep sleep, there was more amyloid beta in their systems after just one night. To make things worse, amyloid-beta plaques build up in the area of the brain that triggers deep sleep, creating a cascade effect: the poorer our sleep quality, the harder it is for the body to flush out amyloid beta, the more amyloid beta there is in the brain, and the less able we are to sleep.

I report all this not to frighten you, but as a reminder of the importance of prioritising sleep and dealing with any sleep-related issues.

My age-well mantra

Remember your dreams! I quickly make a mental note of the dreams I remember when I wake up (however weird they might be). Memory expert Jim Kwik believes this practice helps to boost memory, making it more efficient during the day.

2 Get enough sleep (easier said than done)

Now that you understand your brain's spring-cleaning process while you're asleep, can you name anything that's more important than getting some shut-eye? I thought not. Yet we constantly deprive ourselves of sleep. This week I need you to review your schedule and habits around sleep. If you're not getting enough sleep, what are you prioritising instead?

Let's be clear: sleep deprivation and insomnia are two different things. We deprive ourselves of sleep by not spending enough time in bed, by not having an effective routine for sleep, or by sabotaging our body's attempts to get us to sleep. Insomnia, on the other hand, is a clinical disorder, often related to anxiety, resulting in the brain firing up at night, never allowing the body a break from the adrenalin and cortisol needed to keep it awake during the day. Anxiety, stress and depression are some of the most common causes of chronic insomnia. And, of course, having difficulty sleeping can also make those conditions worse. As you address your sleep habits, you first need to be clear on what's causing your sleep issues, if you have them. Are there wider emotional issues that are causing you anxiety? Or are you feeling anxious because of a lack of sleep? The two are often closely intertwined. I would urge you to seek help for anxiety, via your GP.

Let's focus on sleep deprivation. Why aren't you going to bed? What's keeping you up? Spend this week reviewing your behaviour around bedtime and prioritising the simple act of going to bed. Few things are more important.

The simplest daily actions can sabotage your ability to sleep well. Going to bed and getting up at the same time each day, plus allowing enough time for sleep, are critical. And so is establishing habits, particularly during the evening, that will allow you to fall asleep more easily.

We're surrounded by external stimuli that prevent us from shutting down. Our TVs, laptops and phones are always on, always offering us something to stay awake for. Our towns and cities are brightly lit and filled with the sounds of planes, cars, sirens and other people. All of which conspire to rob us of sleep. It's time to fight back against the sleep thieves!

3 Light days and dark evenings

Probably the greatest external threat to good sleep is the topsy-turvy world of light we now live in. We get up in the dark and dive from buses, cars and trains into artificially lit offices. We come home in the dark to homes blazing with harsh overhead lighting and the non-stop gleam of electronic devices. The brightness of daylight and the gloom of evening that ruled the activities of our ancestors have been lost to us, resulting in circadian rhythms so confused that they can't tell morning from night. No wonder we can't sleep.

To reset our circadian rhythms, we need to recreate the light and dark of the natural world. That means seeking natural daylight, particularly in the morning, and reducing our exposure to light in the evening. Ideally, we should get 30–40 minutes of daylight in the mornings. I work this into my commute when I'm going to an office and a dog walk when I'm not (bonus: I get my step count up too). And I'm increasingly conscious of the light in my home in the evening, using dimmer switches to turn down those lights that I can't switch off completely. It does make the house a bit gloomy, and we make sure the stairs are properly lit so that no one falls, but it helps to move the body and brain towards sleep.

There has been much emphasis in recent years on the role of blue light in the global sleep-deprivation epidemic we now face. Daylight is suffused with blue light, which acts as a wake-up call for our brains. These days, however, we're exposed to blue light from the moment we wake until the moment we close our eyes for sleep. It's there, winking at us, from computer screens, tablets, TVs and LED light bulbs. Our body clock gets constant updates from a light-sensitive protein in our eyes, melanopsin, which measures brightness. Melanopsin is most sensitive to . . . guess what? Blue light. Even Kindles and other e-readers can be a problem, as I explain on page 146.

I reduce blue light from my screens in the evening by using a filter (f.lux) on my laptop and the in-built filter on my phone. I also use blue-light-blocking glasses (quite cheap online). It makes everything a bit sepia, but it's worth it.

The latest research points to the role of all light in causing sleeplessness, however. A team at the University of Manchester found that simply switching blue light for yellow light wasn't enough to encourage sleep – it was the amount of light that made the difference.[5] This is a fast-moving field of research and new studies are published all the time. What is clear is that our modern, over-lit lives are seriously damaging our chances of a decent night's sleep.

A note about eye health

Studies suggest that continued exposure to blue light over time can lead to damaged retinal cells, a cause of age-related macular degeneration.

My DNA test revealed that I have a high genetic risk of this condition, so now I'm very conscious of my eye health. I regularly rest my eyes and make sure that I eat lots of green and yellow vegetables to boost my intake of lutein and zeaxanthin – both plant-based antioxidants that protect our eyes. I rest my eyes as much as I can, and use a warm compress filled with flax seeds to help keep them lubricated.

4 Get into a routine

Going to bed, and getting up, at the same time are increasingly important as we age. The second circadian clock I mentioned on page 127 throws our sleep out of whack. If we stay up to binge on Netflix, scroll through social media or work late into the night, we create a double-whammy effect: piling self-inflicted sleep disturbance on top of age-related circadian disruption.

If you do nothing else this week, get into the habit of going to bed and waking up at the same times each day. See what a difference it makes to your sleep patterns and how you feel each day. Getting up and going to bed at the same times anchors our frazzled circadian clocks, giving them a pattern to stick to. It might mean leaving a party early or missing out on a lie-in, but give it a go this week.

Set yourself a regular bedtime by working backwards from

your morning alarm. Most of us need five cycles of sleep, each of which are 90 minutes long. If it takes you about 15 minutes to get to sleep, and you get up at 7am each day, you need to be settling down by 11.15pm, if not before. I get into bed considerably earlier to read and wind down. If you have the flexibility in your schedule, set a bedtime and wake time that feel right to you. You may be a night owl and want to sleep later, or a lark who loves the early morning. See if you can create a schedule that works to these patterns. Around 30 per cent of the population are morning larks, who fare best with an early start, and 30 per cent are night owls. The rest of us are somewhere in the middle. These traits are genetically encoded, and therefore hard to change.

On page 157 you'll find a sleep tracker so that you can monitor when you go to bed, when you wake, how you sleep and how you feel. Keep a note throughout the week and see how it alters as you follow the guidelines in this chapter.

5 Get your sleep environment right

Build a sanctuary With so much external stimuli, we need to design a sleep environment that's a quiet, calm sanctuary. It's not always easy, but we need peace in which to fall – and stay – asleep. Our bedroom should be free from clutter and the objects that keep us awake: TVs, phones, tablets. Keep chargers out of the way, too. In fact, your bedroom should be as free from the modern world as possible. That means blocking out as much light and noise as you can.

Keep it comfy A good, supportive mattress is a must, as are good pillows. It's all about keeping the neck and spine aligned.

If you're buying a new mattress or pillows, research the different types on the market and test them thoroughly before you splash out.

Keep it clean Dust mites can cause allergies and rashes. Vacuum your mattress and replace it every seven years or so. Try to keep dirty laundry, piles of papers and general mess out of the bedroom. Keep the area under your bed clean and tidy. Weirdly, the knowledge that we're surrounded by mess disrupts sleep patterns.

Keep it cool Our sleeping bodies are incredibly sensitive to temperature; even a fraction of a degree warmer or cooler makes a difference. Our body temperature drops as melatonin production rises: it's one of the cues we need to help us to fall asleep. That's why a hot bath or shower (or sauna) can be a useful sleep aid: our body's cooling mechanism reacts to the hot water, and once that mechanism is switched on the body prepares for sleep. And it's also the reason why we sleep badly in overheated, stuffy rooms. Don't pile on layers of bedding; choose lightweight nightwear and open a window when you can. The ideal temperature is around 16°C/60°F.

Keep it quiet Even low-level sound can rouse us from the deep sleep we need so much as we age. How quiet is your bedroom? If you're struggling with noise, check out the sections on silence (page 141) and pink noise (page 151).

Keep it dark On page 133 I described the importance of dark evenings and light mornings to set our circadian rhythms and to help the production of melatonin, the sleep hormone. Dark and light are also critical in our bedrooms. We need true darkness to help get us to sleep, and to keep us there. Our towns and cities are rarely properly dark. We need to block light pollution from our bedrooms, with eye masks, blackout blinds and curtains. Confession: I use all three!

See my Sleep Kit on page 154 for more ideas on how to make your bedroom pro-sleep.

How I make it work – sleeping

The modern world is designed to keep us awake. There's always another episode to binge on Netflix, another email to send, another social media feed to like. If we're awake, we're consuming, and – often – that means spending, too. That's how the 21st-century economy works. Not to mention societal pressures to have everything under control, be busy, be 'on' all the time. Sleep has become an indulgence: it's for wimps. We lionise people who can get by on a few hours' sleep a night and wish we knew their secret.

Sleep also becomes increasingly elusive and more difficult to get as we age. After researching a solution for the best part of a decade, I'm pleased to be able to tell you that I've got the answer to all this. Drum roll, please.

Go to bed!

We've got no chance of getting quality sleep if we don't go to bed, or if we're glued to a screen when we do get under the duvet. Do your health an enormous favour and give yourself the best possible chance of a decent night's sleep by snuggling down.

If you wake in the night, or have trouble sleeping, try one (or all) of these ideas:

- Just stay in bed and rest. Accept that this isn't going to be your best night's sleep and take the opportunity to rest. Stressing about not sleeping is worse than not sleeping.
- Get up and, in low light, do something simple and repetitive – sweep the kitchen floor, dust a few shelves – then go back to bed.
- Read a non-stimulating book: try poetry or a gentle biography.

If you're struggling, see your GP and ask for a referral to a sleep clinic. Sleep is vital. If you're getting plenty of sleep but you still feel tired all the time, it might be a symptom of an underlying condition. Again, speak to your doctor.

The Top 10: sleep well to age well every night

In an ideal world, we'd all have a great night's sleep, every night. The reality is that's unlikely to happen, particularly as we get older. But there are plenty of simple, effective tricks to help us get more shut-eye. Tick each item below when you've accomplished it.

1 Set an alarm at night

We're all familiar with a morning alarm, but what about an evening one? I set an alarm each evening to tell me to turn down the lights and finish what I'm doing, which might be emails or other chores. This goes off at 9.30pm. A second alarm goes off at 10pm telling me to '*Go to bed!*' That means it's time to go through my night-time routine and actually get into bed. I read for a bit and snuggle down by 10.30pm.

☐　Work out what time you want to set your evening alarm each night. It needs to go off at the same time each evening.

2 Be strict on a daily digital detox

I know I'm banging on about this, but our digital, electronic world is one of the roots of the current global sleeplessness epidemic. An evening spent staring at a screen, scrolling through social media or bingeing on box sets disrupts sleep in several ways:

- By shining blue light into our eyes. This is precisely the type of light designed to keep us awake.
- By delivering constant hits of the neurotransmitter dopamine, which stimulates us to seek pleasure.
- By keeping us alert and 'on' just as we should be winding down.

☐　Try a mini digital detox each evening. No screens for at least an hour before bed.

For me, an evening at home usually consists of clearing up the kitchen after dinner/preparing food for the next day and then working or domestic admin in front of a screen. I now do the former before the latter, so I end my evening pottering in the kitchen.

3 Seek silence

Excess noise – from roads, flight paths, city living and electrical devices – reduces life expectancy by up to three years. Noise exposure causes stress, leading to an increase in inflammation, heart attacks and strokes. At night, noise enters our ears, even as we sleep, and passes through the cerebral cortex (the outermost layer of the brain), rousing us enough to increase blood pressure and disturb our circadian rhythms. This week, evaluate how noisy your sleep environment is and what you might be able to do about it. I live on a busy road under the flight path into Heathrow airport. We shifted our bedroom from the front to the back of the house to reduce noise exposure and fitted carpet to deaden the sound. I also sleep with earplugs every night (see my Sleep Kit on page 154 for my favourite type).

☐ This week, try earplugs and see if they help you to sleep better.

4 Use aromatherapy: the three best oils for sleep

Getting to sleep involves all our senses. And drifting off in a beautifully scented room is one of life's great pleasures. A few drops on the pillow is all it takes. Try one or all of these:

☐ **Lavender oil** An ancient herbal remedy, lavender aids sleep and reduces stress. Professor Russell Foster, head of the Sleep and Circadian Neuroscience Institute at Oxford University, explains that scent is a key way to prepare for bed. In an interview with *The Times* he said, 'Many people will have a certain smell, like lavender, that they associate with sleep. It tells the brain, "It's time to sleep."'

☐ **Valerian oil** The root of this tall flowering grass is used in sleep supplements, and the oil is a common ingredient in bedtime herbal teas. In addition to helping you fall asleep faster, valerian oil might improve sleep quality.[6]

☐ **Bergamot oil** The oil of this Mediterranean citrus fruit gives Earl Grey tea its distinctive aroma. It's known for its calming effect and signals that it is time for bed by slowing the heart rate and lowering blood pressure. Plus, it reduces anxiety and stress.[7]

5 Breathing through a broken night

If I'm finding it difficult to get to sleep, or if I wake in the night, I use a breathing exercise to help me nod off. I learnt it from integrative medicine specialist Dr Andrew Weil. He claims that you can fall asleep in a minute using this technique! I think it takes longer, but it does work for me.

Place the tip of your tongue against the ridge of tissue just behind your upper front teeth and keep it there through the entire exercise.

1   Exhale completely through your mouth.
2   Close your mouth and inhale quietly through your nose to a mental count of four.
3   Hold your breath for a count of seven.
4   Exhale completely through your mouth, making a whoosh sound to a count of eight.
5   This is one breath. Now inhale again and repeat stages 1 to 4 three more times for a total of four breaths. Do the whole cycle four times (making 16 breaths in total). **If you feel short of breath, breathe normally!**

6 How to eat to sleep

Most sleep experts suggest eating three hours before bed to allow the body time to digest. I struggle to get home from work in time to follow this schedule, but do the best I can, usually finishing dinner two hours before I settle down. Certain vitamins and minerals aid sleep. If you're on track with your age-well eating plan, you'll be getting a lot of these nutrients already, but here's a quick primer:

☐   Vitamin B6 helps the body to make the vital sleep hormone melatonin. Find it in sunflower seeds, tuna and wild salmon, avocado, chicken, cooked spinach, bananas, potatoes, whole grains and prunes.

☐   Magnesium is a key nutrient for sleep and many women, in particular, are deficient. Find it in almonds, leafy greens, bananas and fish.

☐   Vitamin E appears to help protect the brain from memory loss associated with sleep deprivation. Find it in nuts and seeds, as well as spinach, broccoli, tomatoes, avocado and wheatgerm.

☐ Vitamin B12 helps to regulate the sleep–wake cycle by keeping our circadian rhythms in sync. You find it in meat, dairy, eggs, fish and shellfish, so vegans need to supplement it. If you're taking a supplement, do so in the morning.

7 How not to eat to sleep

A stodgy meal just before bed, heavy with refined carbs and sugar, won't aid sleep. Once melatonin production has begun in the evening, the body struggles to produce enough insulin to deal with blood sugar spiked by a heavy evening meal. The two hormones don't coordinate well.

☐ Try to eat several hours before bedtime so that insulin can do its work before melatonin production kicks in.

☐ Avoid foods containing tyramine, a brain stimulant, in your evening meal:
    aubergine
    chocolate
    fermented/cured foods
    pineapple
    tomato

My age-well mantra

No puds before bed! (Not very often anyway.) I know that a dessert, or even just some dark chocolate, late in the evening affects my sleep, so if I'm going to indulge, I'll do it mid-afternoon.

☐ Disregard the old wives' tale about cheese disrupting sleep: research has found that people eating a small piece of cheese before bed sleep better than those who abstain.

8 How to drink for sleep

I've ditched the afternoon, and especially evening, espresso in favour of my 'camomile espresso'! I particularly like camomile tea before bed: its sedative qualities are attributed to apigenin, an antioxidant that binds to receptors in the brain, decreasing anxiety and helping us sleep. But the problem with drinking lots of liquid in the evening is needing the loo in the middle of the night. I've learnt to make my camomile tea short and strong! I get the herbal benefits without the 2am trip to the loo. Try a small, strong cup of one of these teas, or make a blend, before bed:

☐ Camomile
☐ Valerian root
☐ Passionflower
☐ Lavender

9 How not to drink to sleep

Alcohol might make us feel sleepy, but it negatively affects the quality of sleep. Critical deep sleep becomes elusive, and REM sleep, which helps us to process emotion, is disturbed. No wonder we sometimes feel 'tired and emotional' the morning after the night before!

☐ Keep tabs on your alcohol intake this week: a small glass of wine with an early dinner is fine, but no night-caps please.

Caffeine can stay in the body for many hours after it's consumed. Depending on how quickly you metabolise coffee, even a cup in the afternoon could jeopardise sleep. For most people, caffeine has a half-life of six hours and a quarter-life of 12 hours, so if you have a cup of coffee at midday, a quarter of that cup is still in your system at midnight.

☐ Monitor your caffeine intake and see how it affects your sleep (you can do this using the sleep tracker on page 157).

10 Read a book

When people were given the same story to read on an iPad or in a book, those reading on the iPad reached slow-wave deep sleep 30 minutes later and had less slow-wave sleep overall.[8] It's that pesky blue light again. But just six minutes of reading a physical book reduces stress levels by 60 per cent,[9] and as stress is one of the key sleep disruptors, it's worth a try!

I read a book in bed pretty much every night before I switch off the light. All e-readers, like Kindles, emit small amounts of blue light.[10] If you use one, check yours to see if it has an internal filter. Kindle Fire has a feature called Blue Shade, while Apple products have Night Shift. You might want to consider a stick-on filter for the screen and/or blue-light-blocking glasses for yourself.

☐   Read in bed for a few minutes every night, but nothing too stimulating – a page-turning thriller or gripping murder mystery might not have the right effect.

Sleep tips to boost your week

The daily, and nightly, routine you create for sleep is what will help you to get the rest you need. But you can increase the chances of a good night's sleep with the practices listed below.

Avoid sleeping tablets if you can

Medicating for sleep is one of the most controversial areas of sleep therapy. What's clear is that medicated sleep – sedation, essentially – doesn't bring the same health benefits to the brain as natural sleep. But it's understandable that someone who's desperately sleep deprived will reach out for whatever help is available. It's not for me to advise you about sleeping tablets (that's between you and your GP), but I can tell you that they knock out deep (SWS) sleep and REM sleep, the two types of rest we need to lay down memories and allow the glymphatic system to do its work taking out the trash from the brain. Which, in turn, increases the risk of Alzheimer's. That's not to say that sleep medication *causes* Alzheimer's, but research shows a correlation between increased risk of the disease and the long-term use of sleeping pills such as benzodiazepines.[11]

☐   Talk to your GP about reducing sleeping pill usage if you feel it's right for you.

Weekends are for napping

Recent research from Greece reveals that an afternoon nap reduces blood pressure, thus reducing the risk of heart attacks.[12] It's difficult to make the Mediterranean ideal of a daily siesta a reality in working life, unless you have a very understanding boss, but can you manage a nap at the weekend? Or on holiday? Nappers have less cognitive decline than non-nappers. The optimal duration is 30–60 minutes; any longer is counter-productive.

☐   Can you fit in a nap this weekend?

Have a magnesium bath

The mineral magnesium is essential for bone strength and over 300 biochemical processes in the body, so a deficiency produces myriad symptoms, including insomnia. Research indicates that half the population might be deficient in this sleep mineral. I tried supplements, but my sleep seemed to get worse! A nutritionist suggested I try a bath with magnesium flakes. The evidence that we absorb this mineral transdermally (through the skin) is a little patchy,[13] but I do sleep well after a magnesium bath. Is it relaxing in a warm bath with a book that does it, or the magnesium? I don't know.

☐ Try to make time for a relaxing bath with magnesium flakes this week and see if it works for you.

Good guts = good sleep

The strong connection between the gut and the brain impacts on how well we sleep. Recent research reveals that better sleepers have more diverse microbiomes and vice versa. The study team suggests that there might be ways to improve sleep in the future by manipulating the gut microbiome.[14] Broadcaster and author Tom Bradby believes that kefir (fermented milk, rich in probiotics) has helped him in his well-documented battle with insomnia.

☐ Introduce a little fermented and prebiotic-rich food into your diet, if you haven't already. But eat it during the day, not at night.

Don't fret about a broken night

If there's one thing worse than a broken night, it's fretting about a broken night. The stress of not sleeping has a bigger impact on our health than the lack of sleep itself. If you have had a few bad nights this week, try to ride it out and accept that your sleep is a work in progress. Log it carefully on the sleep tracker on page 157 and see if you can find any patterns or clues as to why you slept badly? What did you eat or drink in the evening? Were you stressed about something before bedtime?

Remember that sleeping eight hours straight is a product of the Industrial Revolution, when workers manned factories and mines for long hours, illuminated by artificial light. Before that, our forebears enjoyed bi-phasic sleep: going to bed when it got dark and then waking in the middle of the night to do chores, eat and chat before going back to sleep again.

☐ This week, if you wake up in the night, try getting up and doing something dull and repetitive, like sweeping, in dim light. You want your bed to be the place where you sleep, not the place you worry about not sleeping.

When to exercise to sleep well

Week 3 was all about exercising to age well. I know how important exercise is, and how hard it can be to fit it in. In the past, experts told us not to exercise at night in case it interfered with sleep. But recent research turns that advice on its head. In fact, it reveals that people who exercise in the evening actually sleep better at night.[15] The researchers found that people who exercised in the evening got an extra 1.3 per cent deep sleep. That's not much, but we now know how vital every minute of deep sleep is.

☐ If you want to exercise in the evenings this week, go ahead. Just don't do vigorous exercise within an hour of bedtime.

What colour is your noise?

It's a weird question, I know. Different noise frequencies are allocated a colour depending on the intensity and distribution of energy. Certain sonic hues have been associated with better-quality sleep.

White noise Sound is referred to as white noise when the energy distribution is equal across the frequencies; for example, a whirring fan, TV static or a humming fridge. As it contains all the frequencies of sound in equal ratios, white noise can mask the sounds that disturb us at night: the neighbour's dog, a police siren, living under a flight path. It's been found to reduce insomnia.[16]

As I'm on a mission to remove all screens from our bedroom, I invested around £45 in a Dohm White Noise Machine. It's a small contraption that makes a sound exactly like an air con filter and blocks the noise of planes, traffic and an occasionally snoring husband.

Pink noise has more low-frequency components than white noise and increases the effectiveness of deep sleep – the most critical part of the sleep cycle for brain health as we age. In a very unscientific study, I've found playing pink noise in my bedroom at night results in a more restful night's sleep. There are lots of pink-noise videos on YouTube: look for one that lasts eight to nine hours and leave it running on an iPad or phone. Make sure that all the other alerts are switched off and that you can't see the light from the screen.

☐ Experiment with pink noise this week and see if it helps you to sleep.

Black noise The Holy Grail for most of us in our noisy lives, black noise refers to an absence of noise all together, which is very hard to achieve. I use earplugs to help make my world a little quieter. There's more about them in my Sleep Kit.

Meditate and be mindful

A calm, clear mind is the greatest sleep aid there is. You'll learn more about the power of meditation to help us age well next week, but a few minutes of mindfulness can make a huge difference to how well we sleep. Research on a group of sixty-somethings found that those who practised mindful meditation improved their sleep quality more than a group who focused on sleep hygiene (the term used to refer to creating the right routine and environment for sleep), although both groups benefited from the intervention.[17] The breathing exercise on page 142 is a form of meditation, focusing on the breath and counting.

☐ Mindfulness meditation involves simply paying attention to your body – and nothing else. Try it this week when you get into bed.

☐ Become more aware of the sound of your breath or the feeling of the mattress underneath you, for example. If your thoughts wander to your to-do list or the neighbour's dog barking in the garden, just observe that and try to steer yourself back to being mindful without judging yourself.

... and relax

If meditation isn't for you, or you're struggling to get to sleep, try progressive muscle relaxation. It's a simple system of tensing and relaxing all the muscles in the body, a little like the one you may have tried last week on your commute (see page 108), but in reverse.

- It takes 10 to 15 minutes to work slowly through the whole body. Focus on each muscle group in your body, tensing the muscles for a few seconds and then slowly relaxing them over the course of 20 to 30 seconds.
- Start with your head and face, scrunching up your features and wrinkling your brow, then relax all the muscles at once. Bring your shoulders up to your ears, then relax. Work your way through your arms, chest and abs, back, hips and buttocks, legs and feet. Finish by curling and uncurling your toes.

☐ Try progressive muscle relaxation for a few nights this week.

If all else fails, eat ice cream

Not just any ice cream, of course: my sleepy-time ice cream has been a hit on agewellproject.com so I'm sharing it with you here because it's packed with ingredients that aid sleep. Cherries, bananas, honey and yogurt all deliver sleep-enhancing nutrition, and it occurred to me that, together, they would make a rather delicious ice cream.

Sleepy-Time Ice Cream

Serves 4
500g plain Greek yogurt
2 ripe bananas
2 tbsp honey (or to taste)*
1 tbsp almond butter, plus extra to serve
150g (stoned weight) cherries (fresh or frozen), roughly chopped

Blend the yogurt, bananas, honey and almond butter in a food processor. Stir the cherries into the yogurt mixture. Scrape into a freezer-proof container and freeze for two hours or until firm. Allow to soften slightly before serving. Drizzle with a little almond butter and serve.

*The freezing process reduces our perception of flavour, so I make sure that the mixture is slightly sweeter at room temperature than I intend it to be when it's frozen.

How to make it work – my Sleep Kit

Tick any of the following that you need, or want, to buy

- ☐ Good-quality supportive pillows
- ☐ Silk eye mask
- ☐ Mack's ultrasoft earplugs
- ☐ Pink/white noise generator
- ☐ Enjoyable, but not too gripping, novel or a book of poetry
- ☐ Essential oils – lavender, valerian, bergamot
- ☐ Herbal tea – camomile, valerian root, passionflower, lavender
- ☐ Black-out blinds
- ☐ Black-out lined curtains
- ☐ Blue-light-blocking filters
- ☐ Blue-light-blocking glasses
- ☐ Magnesium flakes for the bath

My age-well mantra

Have eye mask and earplugs, will travel. If I'm going away, these are the first things I pack.

My wind-down routine

This is what I aim to do to prepare myself for sleep. Sometimes my evenings don't go according to plan, but I do my best!

Time	Action
9pm	Dim the lights in the house so that the brain prepares for sleep, and draw blackout curtains and blinds. If I can stop looking at a screen now, I will.
9.30pm	First alarm goes: I switch off my screens, if I haven't done so already. I make a small, well-brewed cup of camomile tea, and I might have a magnesium bath, or just potter for a bit, preparing breakfast for the next morning.
10pm	Second alarm goes. I get ready for bed.
10.15pm	In bed with a book and a few drops of essential oil on my pillow.
10.30pm	Lights out, noise machine on, eye mask on, earplugs in. A few moments of mindfulness and slow breathing before (hopefully) I nod off.

Your wind-down routine

What's going to make you feel prepared for sleep? And what time are you going to do it? Use the chart below to work out a realistic wind-down routine for yourself.

Time	Action

Your sleep tracker

Use this tracker to monitor your sleep for a week. Keep a careful note of anything that might disrupt your sleep, like caffeine, alcohol or stress. You should start to see patterns emerge and get a better sense of what impacts your sleep quality.

Night	Caffeine and alcohol intake, stress levels	Time went to bed	Time woke up	Quality of sleep	How you felt the day after
Monday					
Tuesday					
Wednesday					
Thursday					
Friday					
Saturday					
Sunday					

Your personal age-well plan – sleep

Review your sleep tracker and what you've achieved this week: how have you changed your sleeping patterns? What's worked? What hasn't? What's been hardest? What's been easiest? How well have you been sleeping? Which actions worked best for you?

I've listed the key actions again here to remind you. Tick the strategies that have worked well for you. There's a line for notes and reminders too.

☐   Set an alarm at night.

☐   Create a daily digital detox.

☐   Make your sleep environment as quiet as possible.

☐   Try aromatherapy for sleep.

☐   Practise the breathing exercise if you can't sleep.

☐   Review your diet: include food and drinks to help you sleep; eliminate those that don't help.

☐   Get 30–40 minutes of daylight each day.

☐   Turn the lights down in the evening and make your bed-
    room as dark as possible

☐   Read before bed.

☐   Weekend nap.

☐   Magnesium bath.

☐   Mindfulness meditation.

Set your intentions for the future – sleep

Based on the tick list you've just created, write out your sleep
intentions for your own age-well plan; for example, *Every day I
will start a digital detox at 9.30pm, get 30 minutes of daylight
each morning and read in bed.* These intentions will create a list
of good age-well habits that will last a lifetime.

Refer back to your age-well goals, personalised health plan, and age-well eating and moving plans from the last three weeks. Have you been able to keep eating and moving to age well this week? Write out your *purpose* again here to help you remember it:

DR SCOTT CAIRNEY OF THE PSYCHOLOGY DEPARTMENT AT THE UNIVERSITY OF YORK

'Maximise your memory when you sleep'

Scott Cairney is the Medical Research Council's career development fellow and an assistant professor in the Psychology Department at the University of York, specialising in sleep and memory.

The relationship between memory loss and sleep deprivation is complex, but Scott suggests that we should focus on two points: how the simple act of being awake for too long impacts brain function, and how lack of sleep means that we lose the opportunity to process memories. He explains, 'As we go about our day, we're exposed to a wide range of information that can "interfere" with memories of previous experiences.' The longer we're awake, the greater the scope for this overload of information. While we sleep, we consolidate memories, so if we're not sleeping enough, those memories aren't being laid down. 'So, when we're not sleeping, we're not only widening the scope for memory loss via interference, but we're also not getting the crucial sleep we need to prevent this interference from taking place.' A double whammy, in other words.

Learning about the role of slow-wave sleep (SWS) in ageing well has been a revelation to me, so I'm keen to find out from Scott if it's possible to improve it. He explains, 'Given the importance of SWS for memory, optimising it is something that scientists have been trying to figure out for a while. Some earlier work showed that it is possible to stimulate SWS using transcranial direct-current stimulation, but this has been difficult to replicate.'

Scott doesn't pull any punches about the relationship between poor sleep and ageing. 'Unfortunately, as we age, our slow-wave sleep declines. Given the links between SWS and various aspects of cognition and physical health, this might partly explain why we become more prone to illness as we get older. For example, SWS has been linked to glucose metabolism, and young adults deprived of SWS have been shown to become pre-diabetic, temporarily.'

Again, Scott believes that there are two interlinked issues at play here: our slow-wave sleep declines naturally with age, and stresses that arise as we get older are likely to interfere with short-wave sleep duration. 'As we get older, our opportunities for sleep can be affected by various factors (work, stress, children), but we should still try to take steps to ensure that we get the best sleep possible.' And the number-one step to take? 'Routine: our bodies become used to routines, so getting up and going to bed at the same times each day (including weekends) helps to keep our sleep and various other bodily processes in check.'

Scott practices what he preaches, with a regular routine for sleep (and mealtimes, too). 'I find that my biggest problems with sleep have come when I'm stressed, so I try to ensure that I "unplug" myself from work as soon as I get home, such as turning off the email on my phone and not using my laptop. I like to separate my work and home life as much as possible.'

Turning off screens well before bedtime is another key recommendation. And, crucially, Scott believes it's not just about the blue light that they emit, but also about disengaging from the temptation to get on social media and message friends. Something that's all too easy to do!

WEEK 5

How to 'Be'

Now you're eating, exercising and sleeping to age well it's time to add another layer, one that is harder to define. It's easy to focus on the right diet or workout gadget, but how we feel about our lives, how we stimulate our minds and how we interact with others all have a profound impact on how we age too. The mental elements of getting older – social engagement, intellectual stimulation, stress management, practising empathy and cultivating positivity – are as critical as the physical, if not more so.

You're as old as you feel

Staying involved and actively engaged with life is fundamental to healthy longevity. And yet few of us give our mental health the attention it deserves: the highest rates of depression and anxiety in the UK are among those aged 50–59 years.[1] The number of over-fifties experiencing loneliness is set to reach two million by 2025/6. This compares to about 1.4 million in 2016/17 – an increase of almost 50 per cent in ten years.[2] Clearly something needs to change.

We're social animals who have evolved to work as a tribe. Positive interaction with others has a measurable impact on our brain health: the amygdala (the area of the brain that processes emotions and memory) is stimulated by the company of others. The strong social networks enjoyed by SuperAgers might help them stave off mental decline,[3] and Blue Zoners have well-documented friendship groups. In Okinawa, the Japanese Blue Zone, young children are bonded together in small groups known as *moai*. They stay friends (and often see each other every day) for the rest of their lives. Okinawa has the highest percentage of centenarians in the world.

We continue to make new neurons (brain cells) until we die, but only if we keep our brains wiring and firing. Doing that takes as much concerted effort as a new exercise or dietary regime. We need to spend time building a cognitive reserve, the back-up plan for our brain when its power declines. This reserve can mask symptoms of dementia, helping our thoughts navigate past the plaques and tangles of Alzheimer's, just as we might navigate through the back roads when we find ourselves at a roadblock.

Although ageing brings with it many issues, we need to stay positive – we really are as old as we feel. Negativity puts stress on the body by elevating cortisol, which in turn has an impact on heart health, sleep quality, weight and cognition. I've found planning to age well and learning what I can do to help the process extremely empowering – and that helps me to stay positive. I hope you will too.

Assess yourself as you start the week

The questionnaire below will give you an indication of how you're using your mind to age well, your levels of social and intellectual engagement, and how you're managing the stress that can become so debilitating as we age.

Questionnaire: how 'are' you right now?

1　How often do you try something new – a new recipe, walking route, hobby or holiday destination?

2　Do you consider yourself to be very stressed?

3　How do you feel about the ageing process – broadly positive or negative?

4　Do you have a few close friends who you can call if you're having a bad day?

5　Do you have regular social interactions outside the home – from saying hello to the postie to chatting to colleagues, to a hobby or volunteer group?

6　How often do you challenge your brain by learning something new?

7 Do you have some sort of religious or spiritual practice?
   (I include meditation in that.)

8 How often do you do something creative?

9 Do you feel happy?

10 How do you feel about your appearance as you age?

By the end of this week you will:

- Understand the power of novelty.
- Be challenging your brain to learn something new every day.
- Be able to manage stress better.
- Have reached out to more friends.
- Have looked at ways to engage with your community.
- Feel more positive about the ageing process.
- Practise gratitude on a daily basis.
- Laugh more.
- Have considered the role a religious or spiritual practice could have in your life.

The big picture: 'being' – 5 essential lessons

This week we're focusing on engagement – intellectual and social – and your attitude to stress and ageing. This might not be what you expected from this book. But engagement and attitude are critical elements of your age-well plan. Let's focus on why they're so important.

1 Do something new

As we get older, it's easy to get stuck in a rut, following the same patterns that we've followed for years, if not decades. We seek comfort in the familiar. But our ageing brains thrive on newness and novelty. We need to keep challenging ourselves, keeping our brains busy and curious. According to neuroscientist Daniel Levitin, being open to new experiences is one of the most important predictors of successful ageing: 'We just have to be aware and fight the complacency to do the same thing. It's important to surround ourselves with new people – young people – and to try new things. Not dangerous things, but new things.'

Novelty stretches our brains, making them work harder and build new neuro-pathways. We need to stimulate our minds all the time: lifelong learning, volunteering, meeting new people and being creative all fit the bill by encouraging the hippocampus and the amygdala to learn new facts and lay down fresh memories. And while the hippocampus is enjoying all this novelty, its plasticity (the ability to create new connections between neurons) increases, improving memory further.

Learning new things doesn't have to mean tackling a new language or taking up the piano (although both of these are great ways to give your brain a workout). Recent research shows that it's the *variety*, rather than the difficulty, of activities that slows cognitive decline.[4] It can be as simple as trying a new recipe, chatting to a stranger, walking a new route or listening to an informative podcast. SuperAgers read and travel more than the average person, meaning that they constantly expose their brains to new experiences and ideas.

One study found that the parts of the brain linked to learning and memory are activated by new images, as long as they are positive. And you don't have to go far. There's novelty on our doorsteps: no sunset is ever the same, and seasonality makes parks and gardens look different every day. Seek novelty and you'll find it everywhere.

My age-well mantra

What's my new thing? I ask myself this (somewhat ungrammatical) question every day. I try to do something new every day, however small.

2 Manage stress

Stress is the great curse of modern life. We might no longer face the stresses our forebears did – running for our lives from wild animals, for example. But we face stresses of a very different kind.

Stress triggers our fight-or-flight response, leaving us with the stress hormone cortisol coursing through our bodies. That's fine for dealing with short-term stresses – sprinting away from a woolly mammoth, for example – but not for extended periods. Being in this state can severely affect physical and mental health in the long term, deplete immunity and cause sleep deprivation, which causes further stress in a negative spiral.

The ageing process is severely affected by stress: it shortens telomeres and increases the risk of Alzheimer's. Research has shown that women under chronic stress have significantly lower levels of klotho, a hormone that regulates ageing and enhances cognition.[5] This hormone might be the link between chronic stress and reduced life expectancy.

Another study found that stewing over quite minor stresses can cause health issues a decade later.[6] Middle-aged participants who admitted to allowing stress to linger suffered more health issues and chronic illnesses over a ten-year period. Lingering negative emotions weaken the body and render it more susceptible to disease. The research team's advice? Let it go.

That is easier said than done, though, isn't it? We are hardwired to worry and to store up that anxiety. Our brains are designed to think – and overthink – each situation: they keep us safe by evaluating every danger, so we know whether to run or to stand and fight. Sometimes, just acknowledging that this is what our minds are doing can make a difference. Catching a negative or distressing thought, thanking our mind for worrying and keeping us safe, helps to put that thought into perspective. This is the basis of CBT (cognitive behavioural therapy), which teaches us to be more aware of our thoughts and to distance ourselves from the negative ones. When I found the conflicting demands of family, my mum and work overwhelming, my GP sent me on an NHS-funded CBT course. It was extremely helpful.

Stress and depression aren't natural ageing experiences and need to be addressed. If you are stressing about your own health and happiness – or those of loved ones – or financial worries or emotional difficulties, seek support from experts.

3 Be positive about ageing – and grateful for the opportunity

The French boulevardier Maurice Chevalier, is quoted as saying, 'Growing old isn't so terrible – when you consider the alternative.' To have got this far, we've been given an incredible gift. For people born in the UK in 1900, life expectancy was less than 50; now it's over 80. Daily medical breakthroughs enable us to live longer, healthier lives.

A whole new way of thinking about getting older – positive ageing – is blossoming worldwide. The WHO defines positive ageing as 'The process of developing and maintaining the functional ability that enables well-being in older age.' This means that we need to recognise we can make a difference to how we age: a positive attitude to ageing in turn leads to ageing better. Being proactive about ageing – which is exactly what you're doing with your age-well plan – will make the process more successful.

Feeling positive about ageing reduces stress and, recent research shows, reduces the risk of developing dementia. This is true even for people who carry the ApoE4 gene (see page 30).[7] This suggests that positivity is a protective factor and we can cultivate it.

That doesn't mean that it's easy. As we age and become less valued in our society, we struggle to find our place. We have to redefine who we are and identify our purpose. The Okinawans (who seem to have the how-to-'be' element of ageing completely sorted) call their sense of purpose *ikigai*: your reason for getting up in the morning. Find it and you'll live about seven years longer. You've already taken a major step towards positive ageing by cultivating your sense of purpose in Week 1, so remind yourself of that and pat yourself on the back.

Take some time to think through the positives of ageing: the opportunities you have now that perhaps you didn't have when you were younger due to time constraints or other responsibilities, the friendships you have been able to cultivate in recent years or the hobbies and interests you have developed. These are all worth feeling grateful for, as are the simple pleasures of every-day life: delicious food, a brisk walk, a warm home, blue skies, a comfy bed, a good book.

You can create your own gratitude journal on page 192, which will remind yourself about all the things you have to feel positive about as you age.

4 Practise empathy, volunteer, be kind

Helping others, empathising with them and getting involved with our communities all help us to age well, even at a cellular level. People who live in areas with low social cohesion have shorter telomeres, so lack of involvement in our communities literally damages our DNA.

Empathy helps us to imagine why someone might be feeling a certain way, and to be concerned for their welfare. Research shows that the type of empathy we feel alters as we get older: our *cognitive* empathy (the ability to perceive the emotions of another person) declines, but our *emotional* empathy – our ability to share the experience – might increase.[8]

Developing empathy is one of the best ways of enhancing our longevity. Researchers have found that empathetic people really do live longer.[9] The kindest people are simultaneously reducing stress and lowering inflammation.[10] The mind–body connection is that powerful. Looking at things from another person's point of view is the biggest step towards this. Seek opportunities to be kind every day, read books and watch films to understand the perspective of others, look at art to experience not just the piece itself but the artist's creative process.

Volunteering – helping and caring for others – leads to better physical and mental health, and better cognition as we age. Volunteers tracked over a decade by the English Longitudinal Study of Ageing (ELSA) had a lower risk of death than non-volunteers.[11]

In her book *Growing Young*, researcher Marta Zaraska points out that, while following the Mediterranean diet can reduce the risk of dying by 21 per cent, the equivalent figure for the impact of volunteering may be between 22 and 44 per cent. (You can read my interview with Marta at the end of this chapter.) Any comparison of studies from different fields should be treated with caution, but they do give a sense of the importance of helping others as we age.

The age-well benefits of volunteering are extraordinary. The social contact it engenders can have a profound effect on psychological well-being. Being helpful to others gives us immense pleasure, releasing the happiness hormone serotonin and boosting our sense of accomplishment. If you're struggling to find your sense of purpose, volunteering can help you find meaning and direction in life. It also gets us out of the house and moving: older volunteers walk more, have better thinking skills and a lower risk of heart disease.

5 Be sociable

If you want to be happier, have fewer health problems and live longer, build your social networks of family and friends: that's the message from dozens of research papers into the age-well power of our social networks. Conversely, a relative lack of social ties is associated with depression and later-life cognitive decline, as well as with increased mortality. One study found that a lack of strong relationships increased the risk of premature death from all causes by 50 per cent – roughly the same effect as smoking 15 cigarettes a day, and greater than obesity and physical inactivity.[12] Another report was more specific: social interaction with six or seven friends each week reduced mortality risk by 24 per cent.[13]

Researchers at Oxford University described friendship as 'a guarantee for our successful ageing', explaining that 'people embedded in good relationships show, in general, higher levels of happiness, healthier behaviour, a lower incidence of chronic illnesses and lower mortality'.[14] They point to the particular importance of friendship in later life when physical health begins to decline. One possible explanation for this might be found in the sense of control, purpose in life and self-esteem that good networks provide.

It seems that friendship benefits us more as we get older than at any other time in our lives, whereas the benefits of familial relationships on health and well-being is static.[15] The advantages of late adulthood friendship reach beyond psychological well-being. Research shows that social support is also important for maintaining cognitive function and good physical health in old age: cancer and heart attack patients with the largest number of friends make the best recoveries.

Integrate social activity with other age-well practices such as exercising or novelty – workout with a friend or make new friends while trying something new, and you double the benefits.

How I make it work – cultivating happiness

Midlife might be the most anxiety-ridden time of our lives, but happiness is a U-shaped curve, with people reporting the highest levels of joy once they get into their sixties. Older people are so much happier than mid-lifers that one journal asked, 'Is ageing the secret to happiness?' But that's not to underestimate the trials and tribulations of getting older.

Research has found that happy people live longer. In one study, participants were asked how often they experienced the following in the previous week: 'I felt happy, 'I enjoyed life' and 'I felt hope about the future.'[16] We should ask ourselves these three simple questions each week too. The participants who gave positive answers to these questions live longer, healthier lives. Other studies have shown that people who rate themselves as happy are more likely to look after themselves – being active and eating well too – creating a virtuous circle of mental and physical well-being.

Psychologists debate whether it's possible to 'choose' happiness, and there may be many reasons why positive well-being is hard to achieve in our lives at a particular time: ill-health, redundancy, loss and bereavement, for example. But at other times we can cultivate happiness, and that's what I choose to do.

I set an intention to be happy each day, and to experience it rather than chase after it. I know I have a lot to be grateful for and there is so much to appreciate in the world around me. One of the great joys of getting older is that I've come to appreciate simpler ordinary things: sunsets, flowers, smiles. It all seems horribly cheesy as I write it down, but these things do make me happy.

My research for *The Age-Well Project* led me to meditation, which makes me happy on a daily basis. It makes me more resilient too. I'm better able to ride out the ups and downs of life. I also try to follow the Zen Buddhist Golden Rule: 'Do unto others as you would have them do unto you', which can be hard at times, but it does make human interaction more satisfying in the long run!

All the practices and ideas this week cultivate happiness in different ways: when we think about how to 'be' as we get older, being happy is at the heart of it.

The Top 10: 'be' to age well every day

In earlier weeks we concentrated on the physical: the impact that how we eat, move and sleep has on how we age. We focused on small daily habits that can result in big changes. Now we need to create a mental life that matches the physical one, by keeping us stimulated and building new neurons for the rest of our lives.

1 A friend a day

I try to have an interaction with a friend, family member or acquaintance every day. (I don't include work colleagues in this, when I'm in an office.) It's an easy way to reap the benefits of being sociable and having a support network.

I've advocated throughout this book for spending less time

glued to a screen, but social media, used in the right way, helps us connect. The coronavirus lockdown resulted in many of us communicating differently, using platforms such as Facetime, Zoom and WhatsApp in new ways or for the first time. All social media platforms have the power to make us feel like underachievers, comparing our lives/families/holidays to the carefully curated glossiness of others. But if we reframe them as tools for communicating with those who really matter to us, and avoid voyeuristic scrolling, there are some positives.

☐ Try a quick text message, WhatsApp or email to a friend with whom you haven't been in touch for a while.

☐ Post a positive response to a friend's social media message.

2 Try a few moments of mindfulness

Meditation has been one of the most life-enhancing elements of my age-well plan. It's taught me to be more mindful, more present in my life and more connected to the world around me. It's allowed me to handle problems or setbacks more easily by being able to look at them objectively, rather than succumb to stress and feel overwhelmed by events. It's also been shown to support our immune system by dampening the flight-or-fight response.

Mindfulness simply refers to the act of being in the present moment, not distracted by everything around us or the thoughts in our heads. In one study, participants who practised mindfulness for 25 minutes a day were less stressed when presented with difficult tasks after just three days.[17]

☐ Take a few moments to focus on your breath going in

and out. When thoughts pop up, recognise them and let them go, then return your focus to the breath.

☐ Try to practise this, or check out an app such as Headspace or Calm. Most have a free trial period, so you can work out if you like them before committing to a payment scheme.

Three ... or 12 minutes of meditation

One study found that older adults who meditated for 12 minutes a day had reduced biomarkers linked to Alzheimer's and longer telomeres after three months.[18] The participants followed an ancient form of meditation called Kirtan Kriya, a practice in Kundalini yoga. It involves chanting and finger movements, which does feel a bit silly at first, but it quickly becomes a habit. I use a YouTube video as a guide.

☐ Find a quiet place, search for a 12-minute Kirtan Kriya meditation video on YouTube, and have a go.

4 Read a book (again)

Reading isn't just a great way to get to sleep, but also readers live longer, healthier lives. A study at Yale University found that book readers lived for almost two years longer than non-readers![19]

Reading for six minutes a day can reduce stress – one of life's great agers – by up to 68 per cent. That's more than going for a walk, listening to music or sitting down with a cup of tea. Researchers believe that the distraction of being taken into a literary world eases tension in muscles and the heart.

Reading fiction not only increases empathy by expanding our knowledge of the lives of others, but it also allows us to practice empathy by requiring the same kinds of interpretive skills that we activate when engaging with people in real life.

☐   Read on your commute and for a few minutes before you switch the light off at night.

5 Do talk to strangers

Forget what your mum told you: talking to a stranger is the toughest workout we can give our brains. This simple interaction gives the brain so much to process. In an experiment where strangers spoke to each other in a waiting room, all ended up happier as a result.[20] Another experiment found that participants were happier when they treated the barista in a coffee shop like an acquaintance, chatting and making eye contact, than when they bustled through their order, not stopping to make a connection.[21] When you're out and about today:

☐   Greet people.
☐   Pass the time of day.
☐   Engage with other humans.
☐   Don't be embarrassed – you're making the world a better place!

6 Challenge your brain – vocabulary, games and training

Use it or lose it. That's the message from experts who've studied how the brain declines with age. We need to keep our brains working, challenging them to learn new things.

☐ Learn – and use – a new word. Most dictionary websites – I use oed.com – will send you a 'word of the day'. Or pick up a dictionary and open it at a random page!

☐ You don't have to learn in English: try a few words of another language each day and see how quickly you can improve your vocabulary.

☐ Forget your shopping list: if you need to pick up fewer than six items, say them out loud to yourself and then head out. This conscious recall is known as 'declarative memory'.[22]

☐ Flex your working memory by learning phone numbers or do working calculations of your expenditure as you go round the supermarket.

☐ Cognitive training doesn't mean computer-based brain-training games – they only make us better at the game itself. Spend the time doing something that is good for longevity, such as going for a walk. The same goes for sudoku or a crossword: do them if you enjoy them, but not to reduce cognitive decline.

7 Laugh

Laughing helps us to live longer. What could be more positive than that? It reduces the risk of heart disease and stroke, and levels of the pro-inflammatory cytokines that provoke rheumatoid arthritis. Children laugh spontaneously and often; we need to recapture some of that spirit. The body can't tell if our laughs and smiles are genuine, 'so fake it till you feel it' is the mantra here. Seek out an opportunity for a laugh today.

☐ Watch a favourite comedy on TV. Endless reruns of the hits of our youth are available on a channel somewhere.

☐ Visit a comedy club – many have cheap open-mic nights where you might spot a rising star. Laughing together is a highly bonding activity, bringing socialisation benefits.

☐ Keep a joke book in the loo or kitchen for a quick laugh.

☐ Follow funny people on social media (I'll allow you a quick scroll if it's going to make you laugh).

☐ Play word games with friends and family for brain stimulation, laughter and socialising in one go.

8 Be conscientious

One of the key personality traits for a long life is conscientiousness. Luckily, it's something we can all learn. It's a defining feature of SuperAgers and is really about being sensible. In *The Longevity Project*, Professors Friedman and Martin found that 'the most prudent and persistent individuals (as opposed to the happy-go-lucky ones) stayed healthiest and lived the longest'. Neuroscientist Daniel Levitin defines conscientiousness as 'a cluster of traits that has to do with dependability, reliability, doing what you say you'll do, being proactive'. By filling out the questionnaires in this book you are already flexing your conscientiousness muscle. What else could you do?

☐ Make daily plans and use reminder tools or apps to keep you on track.

☐ Schedule time each day or week to deal with small household tasks and admin so that you don't feel overwhelmed.

☐ How you act influences how you feel: if you act as if life is good, you'll feel that way too.

☐ Conscientious people have grit. Don't give up on problems but use them as an opportunity to learn.

9 Express gratitude every day

The grateful life is a longer one. Count your blessings because feeling grateful for something every day, however small, has a positive impact on our longevity. Participants in a research project were divided into three groups and kept a journal every day. One group recorded what were grateful for, the second recorded what irritated them and the third recorded neutral events. After nine weeks, the gratitude group reported a more positive attitude and greater optimism about the future, and they spent more time exercising than the other groups.[23]

☐ Write a list of three things you're grateful for every day and a brief note as to why you think each good thing happened.[24] This focuses your attention on the sources of the good things in your life. Use the gratitude journal on page 192 to get you started.

☐ Take a 'savouring walk'. Walk outside for 20 minutes (hopefully you're doing this daily already to get enough sunlight) and try to notice as many positive things as you can: interesting architecture, the smell of freshly cut grass, a cute cat/dog/child. Acknowledge each one in your mind and try to identify why that thing is pleasurable to you.

☐ Some Christians say grace before a meal. Try a gratitude practice instead, where each person at the table expresses gratitude for something before you all eat. It's very uplifting and even makes grumpy teenagers feel positive!

☐ Remember these words from writer Alice Walker: '"Thank you" is the best prayer that anyone could say. I say that one a lot. Thank you expresses extreme gratitude, humanity, understanding.'

10 Feel good by looking good

Taking care of ourselves, taking pride in our appearance, presents a positive front to the world and, in turn, makes us feel happier. We might resent the wrinkles, grey hair and saggy bits that come with ageing, but there's a lot we can do to make ourselves feel better about them.

☐ A well-put-together outfit, a splash of colour, cared-for hair and skin can all make a difference to our outlook.

☐ Give your wardrobe a good sort out. Get rid of clothes you no longer feel good in.

☐   Try a completely new style or colour combination from the clothes you already have.

☐   There's lots of advice about caring for midlife hair and skin on the agewellproject.com website.

'Being' tips to boost your week

Working on how we are, our state of mind as we age, is a lot of fun! This section gives you a wide range of suggestions for engaging with others, getting creative and bringing 'soul' to the ageing process. You don't have to do them all every week, so pick and choose what's best for you.

Engage with your community

People who live in areas with low social cohesion have more cellular ageing and shorter telomeres, but communities only grow when people get involved. What could you do to get involved with your local community? Think about what might fit your hobbies, skills and interests, and tick one suggestion that you could try, or plan, this week:

☐   Cook at a community kitchen or refuge.

☐   Host a tea party for older adults. The organisation Reengage runs schemes throughout the country (reengage.org.uk) and says that 89 per cent of its volunteers feel happier as a result of getting involved.

☐ Join a clean-up scheme to improve a local canal, river, park or beach.

☐ Train with the Samaritans or Citizens Advice.

☐ Give an afternoon to help at a charity shop or play games with residents at a nearby care home.

☐ Use your professional skills in a voluntary capacity or mentor newcomers to your industry.

☐ What's lacking in your local area? Could you help fill the gap by fundraising or organising an event?

Get spiritual

I'm not suggesting you go and find God. But study after study has shown that active participants in religious practice live longer, healthier lives. The correlation is extraordinary, with frequent attendees of religious services having a 40 per cent chance of living longer, regardless of religious affiliation.[25] Explore what spirituality means to you.

☐ Were you raised in a particular faith? This might be the time to return to it.

☐ ... or find another one that appeals more to you now as an adult.

☐ If you've enjoyed the daily meditation, deepen it at the weekend and try a longer practice.

☐ Find your 'church' in other ways – the shared euphoria of a concert or a sporting event replicates the feel-good factor of a religious service. I've got season tickets at my local football club – nothing beats the thrill of a last-minute winning goal!

Be creative

Creative thinkers live longer, have greater cognitive flexibility and engage more neural networks. You don't have to be a great artist to get creative; you just have to try.

☐ Dig out some paints, buy a cheap canvas and unleash your inner Jackson Pollock, Georgia O'Keeffe or Sonia Delaunay.

☐ Find a weekend crafting workshop near you: crocheting, knitting, glass-making, woodworking and mosaicking are all popular options.

☐ YouTube and Pinterest are full of creative projects: search 'DIY Crafts' for instructions on everything from patchwork cushions to upcycled bird feeders.

☐ You'll learn about beeswax candles in Week 6 and there are lots of kits for homemade versions for sale online. Treat yourself to one and get candle-making!

Challenge yourself

This is the fifth week of your age-well plan, so you've tried many new experiences and introduced many new practices into your days and weeks. Pick one to delve deeper into this week and really challenge yourself. It needs to be tough: something that will build resilience and grit, both key traits of SuperAgers. You might want to:

- ☐ Go completely plant-based for the week.

- ☐ Expand your culinary repertoire by cooking new dishes or in a new style.

- ☐ Extend your daily walk to a proper hike at the weekend.

- ☐ Run further, faster.

- ☐ Stretch your 14-hour daily fast to a 16-hour one.

- ☐ Do a complete digital detox – no screens for 24 hours.

Seek intimacy with a partner or loved one

Physical touch stimulates the release of oxytocin from your brain's pituitary gland, which in turn lowers inflammation. Oxytocin is known as the 'love hormone' because it is triggered when we hug, kiss, cuddle and have sex.

Intimacy isn't (just) about having sex with a partner, however. It's about close relationships in general with family and friends. According to gerontologist Dr David Lipschitz, 'True intimacy, in whatever form, requires understanding, compassion, trust and empathy. In its purest form, it means entering into the life of another and discovering the richness and uniqueness that exist within each person, and together making life even brighter than it was before.'

☐   Consider the role of intimacy in your life this week.

Don't give into stereotypes about ageing

In cultures where elders are respected and the wisdom of age revered, older people live longer, healthier and more fulfilling lives. But in the West, the view of anyone over the age of 45 can be negative. These negative stereotypes affect older adults' cognitive and physical performance and even their recovery from disease.[26]

Unfortunately, when we are stereotyped in a particular way, we end up living out the assumptions made about us. As we focus on how to 'be' this week, bear in mind the stereotyping of older people.

☐   What representations of older people do you see around you?

☐   To what extent do they reflect your experience?

☐   How do you feel about them?

Hum!

If there is one physical key to health and happiness, it might be the vagus nerve. This nerve (or, more accurately, bunch of nerves) connects most of the major organs between the brain and the colon and moderates our fight-or-flight response. It's largely responsible for the brain–body connection, and stimulating it is the single best thing that we can do to reduce stress and age-related inflammation.

The vagus nerve responds to messages from our breath, relaxing heart rate and lowering stress levels when our breathing is slow and calm, and speeding them up when our breathing rate spikes. All of the actions below stimulate the vagus nerve. Try one, or all, of them this week:

☐ Deep, rhythmic breathing (try breathing in for five counts, then out for five counts).

☐ Laughing has a similar effect.

☐ Cold showers. You're doing this already, right? (See page 108.)

☐ Humming. Yes, humming. The vagus nerve is connected to the vocal cords, so humming a tune, or a low 'om', will stimulate it.

My age-well mantra

I hum in the shower! It means that I can power through another age-well action without it taking any extra time.

Plan a 'people I love' party

Recent research has found that people over 55 with a healthy memory are more likely to engage in social activities such as planning and hosting parties.[27] I occasionally host 'people we love but don't see enough of' parties to reconnect with old friends.

It doesn't have to be fancy: ask people to bring a bottle/plate of snacks and throw open your home. I've found that giving guests a fairly long time frame – perhaps between 3pm and 9pm – makes the party more relaxed.

☐   Send out your invitations this week!

Tap yourself young

The thymus gland is known as the body's 'happiness point'. It's also a vital part of the immune system, helping T-cells to circulate. (T-cells are white blood cells that defend the body from potentially deadly pathogens – the T stands for thymus-derived.)

The thymus sits under the upper part of the sternum, between our lungs. It shrinks from puberty onwards, but gentle tapping can stimulate it, which is why gorillas and ancient warriors beat their chests! Learn to tap your thymus for increased energy and vitality, and to boost the immune system:

☐   Make a soft fist with your dominant hand. Give your sternum one light thump, then gently tap the area for about 30 seconds – you should get 60–100 taps done in that time. Try it a few times this week.

Be optimistic

Studies have found that the most optimistic individuals live between 11 and 15 per cent longer, and have a 50–70 per cent greater chance of reaching 85 years old, than their most pessimistic counterparts.[28] Scientists aren't quite sure why this happens, but it could be that optimists are able to regulate their feelings and bounce back from difficulties more easily. Optimists also tend to have healthier habits.

It's possible to train yourself to be optimistic. Cultivate optimism by:

☐ Trying a 'positive lens'. If something's gone badly, look for a way to reframe it in a more positive, or at least less negative, way.

☐ Seek out people in your social circle who are 'radiators' not 'drains'! Spend time with friends who are full of positivity and don't moan all the time. Avoid the office-kitchen moaners – you know who they are.

☐ Limit your exposure to the daily news cycle and don't listen to the news late in the evening. It can get very depressing.

☐ Acknowledge that you can't control everything and don't fret over every situation. Focus on the things you *can* control.

How to make it work – a gratitude journal

Cultivate the protective benefits of positivity by writing down things you feel grateful for.

Research has found that regularly noting feelings of gratitude in a journal leads to increased altruism, which in turn makes us more positive.[29] It's important to create a physical record by writing. It's not enough simply to do this exercise in your head.

How to journal

- Set a time to keep your journal, possibly just before bed.
- For at least one week, write down three things that went well for you during the day, or you felt gratitude for. Note, too, why they were good. It doesn't matter if they were small or large events – a sunny walk is just as gratitude-worthy as a major promotion, for these purposes.
- As you write, give each event a title – for example, *Sunny walk* – then list why you're grateful for it.
- Also write down how this event happened; for example, *I gave myself permission to take an hour off chores/work and go for a walk.*
- Keep focused on the positive. If you have negative thoughts, such as, *That was a waste of time*, refocus your mind on the good feeling that came with the event.

Suggested gratitude journal layout

Day	Events	Why do you feel gratitude?	Why it happened
	1.		
	2.		
	3.		
	1.		
	2.		
	3.		

Repeat for seven days

Your personal age-well plan – how to 'be'

Review what you've achieved this week. What's worked? What hasn't? What's been hardest? What's been easiest? What have you been doing? How do you feel?

I've listed the key actions again here to remind you. Tick the strategies that have worked well for you. There's a line for notes and reminders, too.

☐   Do something new.

☐   Meditate to manage stress.

☐   Daily gratitude, and keep a gratitude journal.

☐   Practise empathy.

☐   Be social, and plan a party.

☐   Cultivate happiness and optimism.

☐   Community engagement.

☐   Do something creative.

☐ Challenge yourself.

☐ Hum.

☐ Challenge your brain.

☐ Tap your thymus.

Set your intentions for the future – to 'be'

Based on the tick list you've just created, write out a list of intentions for how you want to be as you age; for example, *I will contact one friend each day ... hum in the shower ... tap my thymus three times a week*. This will help you to stick to your own age-well plan.

Refer back to your age-well goals, personalised health plan and age-well eating, moving and sleeping plans from the first four weeks. Have you been able to keep eating and moving to age well this week? How well have you been sleeping? Write out your age-well *purpose* again here to help you remember it:

MARTA ZARASKA, SCIENCE WRITER, JOURNALIST AND AUTHOR

'Use friendship, kindness and optimism to help you age well'

Marta Zaraska is the author of *Growing Young: How Friendship, Optimism and Kindness Can Help You Live to 100*.

When Marta began investigating how best to give her young daughter a long and healthy life, she stumbled across research indicating that social relationships could be the key to longevity, rather than, say, the amount of broccoli we eat. Over 600 research papers and 60 scientific interviews later, she's convinced that we might have the balance wrong as we strive to age well.

Marta invites us to imagine Miss A, a health junkie who chooses the gym and shopping for superfoods over spending time on relationships, friends or volunteering; and Mrs B, who is a little overweight, loves cookies but who's engaged with her neighbours, extremely empathetic and is happily married. 'The question is,' says Marta, 'who's healthier? They may be the same, or Mrs B might actually be better off. It's mind-blowing when we consider the way we currently evaluate health.' She believes that we've become so fixated on counting calories, or steps, that we've lost sight of the real priorities. 'I find it wholly satisfying that there's a fairness to life: if you're a very nice person, you'll live longer. And it doesn't require money – that's the nice part.'

Polish-Canadian by heritage, Marta has lived in France for 12 years and has noticed that the French are much less obsessed than we are in the UK with the idea of *what* they eat, and much more obsessed with *whom* they eat with. She urges us to try to do both: eat healthily with friends; run with a pal rather than alone on a treadmill; use mowing the lawn for an elderly neighbour as a workout. Small random acts of kindness like this also improve our psychological well-being and reduce stress.

We're social apes, so being with our tribe is important both psychologically and physiologically. Marta explains, 'The tribe means safety, so our stress axis has evolved to calm when we feel strongly connected to others. Stress goes through the roof when we're lonely.' And we don't just need to be with our tribe; we need to be empathetic towards them, too. She urges us to develop empathy, 'start paying attention to other people, try to look at situations from their point of view. Reading fiction is a great way to become more empathetic.' It helps us understand the lives and thoughts of others, making us more compassionate as a result.

Despite being a busy mum, Marta finds time to meditate or do yoga every day and suggests that we try to do the same. 'Even a little bit is better than nothing; meditation helps us to breathe better and slower, which in turn might lead to longer telomeres. Don't get hung up on different yoga styles – they all work.'

Marta's key message? 'Just do it! We all have a limited amount of time, so we have to choose the things that are most important. It's about priorities: do we really need to spend time searching for the world's best broccoli or should we make time for friends?'

WEEK 6

How to Live

You have reached the final week of your age-well plan – congratulations! In the last five weeks, you've given your body, brain and soul an age-well makeover. You've created daily and weekly action plans which will last for the rest of your life. But I have to sound a note of caution here. However hard we work on our personal health and take responsibility for ageing well ourselves, we don't operate in a vacuum. We live in a busy, toxic world, ill-designed for longevity. How we negotiate that, inside and outside our homes, is vital to our age-well plan.

Ageing in the world around us

Almost every week, it seems, a new research paper is published on the devastating impact of pollution and our environment on our risk of dementia, heart disease and cancer; not to mention how the chemicals that infiltrate our lives affect mental health, skin ageing, gut diversity and much more.

This week we'll be looking at reducing the harmful impact of the outside world on our ageing bodies and minds, and what we can do inside our own homes to help us to age well. We'll reduce the impact of pollution and plastics at home and beyond it, think about car usage and slash the number of toxic chemicals we come into contact with every day. We'll think about the environment we would like to age in, and how we're going to make it happen.

This is also the time to start thinking about how we're going to live in the future, once our six weeks of ageing well together is over. What do you want your age-well future to look like? Where will you age, and with whom? Do you have the financial, familial and social support you need to make your age-well dreams a reality?

Assess yourself as you start the week

This is the moment to think about your interactions with the world around you, to evaluate how you live, and to consider what you'd like your life to look like going forward. This week is all about forward planning, so take a moment to work out where you are now.

Questionnaire: how are you living now?

1   How much do you use your car?

2   When did you last use a map or allow yourself to get lost and navigate your way back?

3   How often do you see a tree in daylight (through a window doesn't count)?

4   How often do you open the windows in your home?

5   Do you use any natural or organic cleaning products?

6   Do you use any natural or organic skincare/ bath products?

7   Do you ever eat organic foods? If so, how much?

8   Have you (and your partner) considered your future?

9   What about work? Are you still working?

10 Are you ready for an age-well life?

By the end of this week you will:

- Have re-thought your relationship with your car and be driving less.
- Be spending more time outdoors.

- Have overhauled the cleaning products in your home.
- Have considered your skincare and bath products.
- Understand the importance of the Dirty Dozen and the Clean 15.
- Have reviewed your finances.
- Be discussing your plans for an age-well future.
- Have considered the role of work in your life.
- Be able to look ahead with excitement!

The big picture: an age-well life – 5 essential lessons

This week we take your age-well plan out into the world, looking at how pollution, chemicals and our environment affect how we age; and we examine what that means for the choices you make about your future.

1 Why the air we breathe is killing us – outdoor pollution

No, I'm not exaggerating. The WHO has declared air pollution a global health emergency and blames it for one-third of all deaths from stroke, heart disease and lung cancer. Air pollution is not just something affecting the world's busiest streets; more than 90 per cent of the global population endure toxic air. A bigger killer than tobacco, 8.8 million early deaths are attributable to the air we breathe.

Almost every cell in our bodies is affected by air pollution, with recent research showing head-to-toe harm, that includes our lungs, skin, bones and brains.[1] The damage is caused in myriad ways, triggering acute responses, such as lung infections and heart attacks, and chronic conditions, including dementia and osteoporosis. There was a close correlation between Covid-19 and pollution across Europe in spring 2020, with almost 80 per cent of deaths from the virus in the most polluted areas of Germany, Italy, France and Spain.[2] Exposure to environmental toxins causes our mitochondria to misfire and our telomeres to shorten.[3] One study associated increased exposure to air pollution with lower levels of verbal learning, logical memory and executive function in middle-aged and older adults.[4] Some of these health issues occur as a direct response to ultra-fine particles finding their way to our organs. Others occur as a result of inflammation throughout the body in response to toxic air.

These problems are caused by a cocktail of airborne pollutants from a variety of sources, including petrol and diesel exhausts, aircraft fumes, pesticides, industrial emissions and animal husbandry. Below is a list of the most dangerous pollutants:

- **Particulate matter** (PM) is a general term for the particles which form when gases emitted by cars and factories react together in the air. It's classified by size of the particle. Larger particles, such as the coarse PM10, are visible to the naked eye and form the dust haze, or smog, so familiar in cities. These larger particles affect our upper respiratory tract and mucous membranes, but they can't enter the bloodstream. Motes smaller than PM2.5 (1/40th of a millimetre) enter the bloodstream, and the brain, and are linked to heart disease, dementia and asthma. It is believed that they contribute to 29,000 deaths due to respiratory problems in the UK each year.
- **Nitrogen dioxide** (NO_2), a by-product of the combustion of fossil fuels, can penetrate deep into the lungs. It is linked to bronchial and respiratory diseases.

- **Ozone,** the result of pollutants from cars and industry reacting in the presence of sunlight, is linked to respiratory failure and premature death.
- **Sulfur dioxide,** released into the air by the burning of coal and oil in power plants, is highly soluble and causes damage to the upper respiratory airways and skin.
- **Carbon monoxide,** another by-product of fossil-fuel combustion, can be emitted by household appliances like boilers and heaters. It reduces the amount of oxygen carried around the body by the haemoglobin in red blood cells. This has been linked to heart problems.

People with raised exposure to PM2.5 increase their dementia risk,[5] particularly if they carry, as I do, the ApoE4 gene. I live on a main road, and under the flight path into London's Heathrow Airport. Fifty-year-olds in polluted London have the cognitive abilities of 60-year-olds in the cleaner air of Plymouth.

There's no escaping the fact that I'm exposed to a deadly cocktail every day. But I remain upbeat about it, knowing that there are some things I can do to mitigate my risk, and accepting that there are some things I can't change.

2 What's happening in your home?

Sadly, our homes aren't always the safe havens we hope them to be. The modern home often contains an even more toxic combination of chemicals than our dirty, polluted streets. It's been estimated that we spend about 90 per cent of our time indoors, in private and public spaces, meaning that indoor air quality (IAQ) might be far more important to our health than outdoor air quality.[6]

Toxic air in our homes is a potent brew of pollutants, which have infiltrated from outside, and contaminants, which originate inside, such as smoke from burning fuels and candles, emissions from building materials and furnishings, central heating and cooling systems, electronic equipment, household cleaning products and pets. Then there are the toxins produced by our own activities: from smoking to spraying perfume to crafts.

An analysis of the composition of dust in the average home identified 45 toxic chemicals. Flame retardants, fragrances and phthalates (a group of chemical binding agents used in everything from cleaning products to food packaging to lipstick) were found in at least 90 per cent of samples.[7] These have been linked to an increased risk of breast cancer, type-2 diabetes, obesity and hormonal issues.

On a daily basis we spray chemicals around our homes to keep them clean and sweet smelling, with little thought for what's in them. We fill our kitchens with plastics and our bathrooms with more pollutants. We wash and moisturise our bodies with further chemicals. None of these, used individually and according to the manufacturer's instructions, is likely to cause health problems. There's no clear-cut answer to the impact of chemicals and pollutants on our homes, no formula that pinpoints the moment at which they become toxic to us.

Our response to chemical build-up is as individual as we are, so there's much uncertainty about which chemicals cause these problems, and at what concentration. Here's just one example published early in 2020: in this particular study, participants with the highest exposure to a class of pesticides called pyrethroids had three times the risk of death from cardiovascular disease, compared to those with the lowest exposure.[8] Few of us have high exposure to these insecticides (unless we work in the crop spraying business), but many of us are exposed to them at a low level via household insecticides such as moth sprays, pet shampoos and mosquito repellent. At what point do they start to become toxic? My response might be different from yours. And both our responses will be affected by the other chemicals we come into contact with. Research into this complex field is still at an early stage. What is clear, however, is that we need to reduce our exposure to chemicals in our homes, as our resilience and tolerance diminish with age.

3 Plastic – not fantastic

In 2017 it was estimated that around 8.3 billion tonnes of plastic had been produced worldwide in the 70 years since it was first industrially manufactured.[9] Just 9 per cent of this total had been recycled and 12 per cent incinerated, leaving 79 per cent to accumulate in landfill or elsewhere in the natural environment.

Like us, plastics age. As they degrade they shed microplastics, invisible fibres that now effectively coat our planet, turning oceans into plastic soup, impacting marine life, infiltrating our water systems and floating in the air we breathe. Microplastics have been found at the top of French mountains and at the bottom of the deepest oceans.

Humans are not immune from the impact of microplastics. A recent study estimated that the average American ingests between 39,000 and 52,000 particles of plastic. That figure rises to 74,000 and 121,000 when inhalation of air-borne microplastics is taken into account.[10] Even more worryingly, the research team considers these numbers to be underestimates.

We drink plastic when we imbibe water (particularly if it's from a plastic bottle), we eat it when we consume seafood or foods that have been packaged in plastic, and we inhale it when we breathe. But is it actually doing us any harm as we age?

The jury's still out on the exact effects of plastics on our health. Some chemicals found in plastics, such as bisphenols and phthalates (them again) disrupt hormones. And studies on zebrafish and mice have linked microplastic intake to mutations in gut microbiota, increased inflammation and oxidative stress,[11] three of the key markers for ageing. It doesn't sound good, does it?

Where it goes from here, we don't know. Early research on human cells in vitro suggests that the inflammatory response to microplastics seen in animals might well translate to humans.[12] There's clearly a lot more research to be done, but in the meantime we have to do all we can to reduce our use of plastics.

4 Noise pollution

Pollution comes in many different forms, not just from chemicals and plastics. The traffic that poisons our air also impacts our hearing. We might hardly be aware of it, but we're constantly exposed to noise: traffic, planes, building work, machinery, other people's music ... the list goes on. This aural barrage has been linked to hearing loss, sleep disturbance, heart disease, obesity, tinnitus, dementia and diabetes. All of which we work so hard to avoid as we age.

The WHO declared noise pollution to be the second largest environmental threat to health in the EU, after air pollution. And while Britain might no longer be part of the EU, the problem remains. The WHO goes on to report that traffic noise alone results in an annual loss of 'at least one million healthy years of life' across Western Europe each year.[13]

Although researchers often find it difficult to differentiate between the effects of air pollution and noise pollution generated by traffic, when a team from Imperial College London adjusted their research they found that biomarkers linked to stress and inflammation increased further due to noise. They found that an increase in noise of just five decibels (literally the sound of a pin dropping) increased blood sugar (a precursor to diabetes).[14] In a further study, the same research team also found a possible association between road traffic noise and ischaemic heart disease.[15]

Even if we think we block out noise, it might still affect our heart rate, blood pressure and stress levels. And while we sleep, noise percolates our consciousness, lifting us out of the deep sleep that's so vital as we age. This, in turn, disturbs our circadian rhythms, resulting in us feeling unrested during the day.

Hearing loss is one of three chronic conditions that most reduce quality of life for the elderly, along with failing eyesight and backache. It's believed that seven million Britons could benefit from hearing aids, but only two million use them. When did you last have your hearing tested? Ask your GP to refer you for tests if you have concerns. Wearing a hearing aid in mid- and later life can slow brain ageing and fend off dementia – I bet you're thinking about that test now, aren't you?

5 When all else fails, seek out green and blue space

How well we age is directly affected by how much time we are able to spend in nature. Across the world, those living with more green space report better general health and suffer less cognitive decline.

For one research paper, 6,500 people in the UK – aged 45 to 68 – underwent extensive cognitive testing over a period of ten years. The results were then analysed and correlated with satellite pictures showing the amount of green space in their neighbourhoods. Those living with abundant greenery had slower cognitive decline than those who lived in more urban areas. Although the difference in cognitive decline was small (4.6 per cent), the correlation between green spaces and slower cognitive decline was more marked among women.

Further research across the world has correlated time spent close to nature with significant and wide-ranging health benefits, including reduced risk of type-2 diabetes, cardiovascular disease, premature death, high blood pressure and stress. Increased sleep duration was also reported by those living with more green space.

The Japanese have developed the idea of *shinrin yoku*, literally 'forest bathing', which is believed to boost immunity and reduce stress. Researchers aren't really sure why this happens. Is it the exposure to bacteria in the soil that could reduce inflammation? Is it the immune-boosting phytoncides that are released by trees? Is it the opportunity for physical exercise provided by green space? Gardening has a similar impact.

A note on gardening

Gardeners live up to 14 years longer than non-gardeners and are less stressed. Why? It's the combination of physical exercise, fresh air, green space, vitamin D, exposure to gut-boosting bacteria in the soil and – potentially – the benefits of home-grown vegetables.

If green space is good for us, it might transpire that blue space – landscapes containing water – could be even better. Research in this area is still at an early stage but an analysis of 33 studies concluded that landscapes containing water offer 'potential health benefits ... mainly with respect to mental health and well-being'.[16] A further study involving data from nearly 26,000 people found that those living within a kilometre of England's coastline, particularly those in the lowest-earning households, had better mental health than those living inland.

How I make it work – see a tree, in daylight

'See a tree' combines so many of the age-well habits you're developing: being outdoors in daylight, exercise from walking, a chance to savour, and even one lonely tree provides us with a little green space. Hence, I've added seeing a tree to my daily age-well to-do list. It doesn't take any more time than my morning walk, but it adds focus to my journey.

Contact with nature reduces stress, we know, and recent research has sought to quantify the specifics of how long, and how often, we need to be in nature for it to have a measurable impact on our health. The results show that 20 minutes makes a huge difference, but a little longer – up to 30 minutes – is best. The research team calls these short bursts of outside time 'nature pills' and they hope that, in the future, doctors will prescribe them to combat stress.[17] That's the kind of age-well medicine I like.

The 'in daylight' element of this age-well activity is important, too. Natural light has been found to increase concentration in students and productivity in office workers, as well as reducing the duration of patients' hospital stays. It boosts serotonin, the 'happiness hormone', and sleep quality by keeping our circadian clocks ticking accurately. Daylight provides more than bone-boosting vitamin D. It boosts immunity by powering up T-cells, increasing their capacity to fight off infection, and helps to transfer nitric oxide from the skin to the circulatory system, thereby reducing blood pressure. Time to get outside!

The Top 10: live to age well every day

The world around us is complicated, noisy and dirty – we know that. But there are simple things that we can do each day to reduce the environment's impact on our ability to age well. The format is slightly different this week, with more emphasis on long-term projects, such as switching to safer cleaning products and reducing pesticide exposure, rather than daily habits.

1 Avoid busy streets – and your car

When we started the Age-Well Project, I didn't own a car. I walked a lot, took buses and used car clubs. As my children got older and needed ferrying further afield, being carless became impractical for us. But I try to use it as little as I can.

When we sit in cars we are more exposed to toxins from air pollution than at any other time. Overall air quality can be 15 times worse inside vehicles than on the pavement, and sitting in traffic jams makes the situation even worse, with pollution levels inside cars rising by 40 per cent.[18] Researchers suggest closing car windows and setting the fan to recirculate air in bad traffic.

☐ How can you reduce your car usage this week?

☐ If you have to use your car, make use of the fan when in traffic jams.

☐ If you're walking on busy highways, keep as far from the road as you can, and if you can walk on a side street, do. Pollution is 10 per cent worse on the road side of a pavement than on the building side.

2 Plan walking routes and use a map

Avoid your car and you'll walk more. You'll log more steps in a day and also give your memory a workout, provided you ditch Google Maps and rely on a paper map, or your own brain, instead. Some neuroscientists believe our 'place' cells are dying off because we're no longer using them to navigate. The hippocampus, which lays down memories, evolved for geo-navigation – to help us remember where we are going, where dangers lie and where we might find food. Navigation builds resilience in the hippocampus and the entorhinal cortex, the region of the brain where Alzheimer's might begin.

☐ Plan a route, follow a map or just go for a wander to exercise your geonavigational skills. London cabbies who have successfully completed 'the knowledge', thus committing the city's highways and back routes to memory, have bigger hippocampi than the average citizen.

☐ Go further afield, plan a hike somewhere you don't know. And use a paper map, rather than the one on your phone.

☐ Don't forget to see a tree on your way!

3 Eat to beat pollution

Early research suggests that eating the right foods might help us to lower pollution-related inflammation in our bodies. Our friend the Mediterranean diet helps,[19] and eating two large handfuls of cruciferous (brassica) vegetables a day (broccoli, cabbage, cauliflower, kale) is associated with a 20 per cent reduced risk of dying from pollution-related illness.

Vitamin D might protect our airways from inflammation caused by particulate matter (see page 36 for more on supplementation), but many other nutrients appear to play a role in helping our lungs fight the good fight against air pollution. Try to eat some or all of these this week:

☐ **Vitamin C** Kiwi fruit, citrus fruit, peppers
☐ **Carotenoids** Carrot, sweet potato, squash, watermelon
☐ **Vitamin E** Avocado, nuts
☐ **Omega-3 fatty acids** Oily fish, walnuts, flax seeds, chia seeds and edamame
☐ **Choline** Eggs, liver, peanuts, tofu, broccoli
☐ **B vitamins** Whole grains, wheatgerm, leafy greens, liver, eggs
☐ **Genistein**[20] Soya and soya products such as tempeh and tofu

4 Rethink your cleaning products – what to ditch

The cleaning products we use daily in our homes add to the build-up of toxins around us. Some release harmful volatile organic compounds (VOCs) into the air, contributing to up to half of VOCs found in the atmosphere. Some VOCs have been linked to cancer, while others react with pollutants in the atmosphere to cause irritation to the eyes, nose and throat, and damage to the liver, kidneys and the central nervous system. These compounds break down into the air pollutant PM2.5, which cause myriad health problems.

In addition, a huge number of household items – including air fresheners, hand sanitisers, detergents and deodorants – are perfumed with a cocktail of ingredients. These scents also emit potentially toxic VOCs.[21]

It's easy to think: *Oh, but I only use a dollop of detergent in the washing machine and a smidge of shampoo when I wash my hair.* But the effects are both cumulative and dependent on individual health issues. The choices you make at this point are individual, too. I've ditched the following products – see if you can, too:

☐ **Bleach** We know not to drink the stuff, but just inhaling the fumes is enough to damage the respiratory system. Regular use has been linked to increased risk of developing chronic obstructive pulmonary disease (COPD).

☐ **All-purpose sprays and window/glass sprays** Using cleaning sprays daily for 10–20 years can impact lung function. In one study the effect was comparable to smoking a packet of cigarettes a day for the same amount of time.[22]

☐ **Oven cleaner** They may be super-efficient, but most oven cleaners contain lye (sodium hydroxide), which is extremely corrosive.

☐ **Floor soap/cleaner** This is the biggest area in the kitchen to keep clean and I don't want to cover it in toxins.

My age-well mantra

Do I need to use this product? There's often a lower-tox alternative.

5 Rethink your cleaning products – what to use

Having ditched some of the most chemical-laden cleaning products in my home, I now either make my own or buy more environmentally friendly versions. Commercially available green cleaning products are, of course, more expensive than the regular ones. I'll leave it up to you to decide where you spend your money (although turn to Appendix IV on page 273 for my favourite brands). I save a lot by making some of my own cleaning products, so I don't mind splashing out more on the items I don't make, such as washing-up liquid.

There's something deeply satisfying about making your own – treat it like a weekend craft project – and knowing that you're benefiting your own health as well as that of the planet. It gives a sense of purpose to the simple act of looking after your home, which doesn't come from a plastic spray packed with chemicals.

☐ Put together a small kit of ingredients from which you can make a few simple home-cleaning products.

☐ Turn to Appendix IV on page 273 for my cleaning product ingredients and recipes. I also use coconut or bamboo cloths (to reduce shedding of plastic micro-fibres) and water (plus elbow grease, as my mother used to say!).

6 Open your windows

Our fuel-efficient and well-sealed homes leave little room for ventilation. The drive to reduce energy costs – a good thing, obviously – allows the build-up of a range of pollutants, which makes airing our homes properly a vital daily activity. This can also help to reduce the condensation that creates damp and mould. Our immune and respiratory systems are impacted by damp, and the mould and bacteria that come with it.

☐ Opening windows for just 15 minutes a day is enough to air your home and reduce the levels of pollutants.

☐ Consider an air purifier. I haven't invested (yet) – the best ones cost up to £500. If you're tempted, make sure you buy one that has a HEPA (high-efficiency particulate air) filter to deal with particulate matter (PM) and an activated carbon filter to deal with VOCs. There's a detailed post on the best purifiers at agewellproject.com/air-purifiers/.

7 The age-well skin you're in

If avoiding harsh chemicals in our homes helps us to age well, avoiding them on our bodies is even more important. You'll have heard this before, but our skin is our largest organ of detoxification. It makes sense that if we plaster it with nasties, it's unlikely to function well.[23] And, like everything else, our skin's resilience diminishes with age. It gets thinner and loses the collagen that gave it a youthful bounce.

Our skin is constantly under assault, not just from ageing but also from the sun, diet, stress, tobacco smoke, lack of sleep, temperature fluctuations and, increasingly, pollution.[24] Air pollution has been found to create age spots, increase wrinkles and deplete antioxidants from the skin. We need to keep our skin protected, without adding to its toxic load. I've swapped out big-name brands for these – consider if you'd like to do the same:

☐ **Skincare and bath products** Seek out organic skincare products that are free from parabens (linked to breast cancer) and phthalates. Good brands to check out include Antipodes, Neal's Yard, Green People, Whamisa, Korres, Lyonsleaf and Organic Surge.

☐ **Eye make-up remover** Use coconut oil! It works perfectly. I rub a tiny drop onto a washable cotton pad and wipe away – it's simple, cheap and effective.

☐ **Body scrub** I make my own: mix organic sunflower oil or coconut oil, a large handful of regular table salt and a couple of drops of lavender oil. Store it in a sealed jar in the shower and use it a couple of times a week.

☐ **Sunscreen** Although vital, suncreams and lotions inhibit the skin's production of vitamin D and nitric oxide. I like Dr Weller's Sunwell range, which allows the skin to generate these natural compounds.

☐ **Deodorant** I haven't used a regular deodorant since I breast-fed my first daughter nearly 20 years ago. Instead, I use a salt crystal stick and a natural citrus spray (I like the Weleda brand).

8 A bad smell? Scented candles

I love a scented candle as much, if not more, than the next woman. But many candles, air fresheners and melts are little bombs of toxicity that don't deserve a place in our age-well homes. Candles are particularly problematic because, obviously, they burn. Many contain perfumes that are usually harmless, but which, when ignited, mix with ozone in the air to produce the carcinogen formaldehyde. One candle in a well-ventilated home is unlikely to cause a problem. But when we keep our houses hermetically sealed, burn multiple candles and add other formaldehyde-producing items (the gas is given off by some older types of furniture and flooring, for example), levels build up.

A burning candle also releases particulate matter (PM) and volatile organic compounds. Paraffin candles are popular, as they diffuse scent well, but they can also release VOCs, including carcinogens such as benzene and toluene, into the air.[25] Unscented beeswax candles release comparatively little smoke but do emit some PM particles.

The biggest problem with burning candles at home might be the soot they give off when blown out, and soot is probably the biggest polluter of all. What's the best way to put out a candle? Don't blow, dip! Push the wick into the pool of wax that's formed around it, then lift it out. There are tools available to do this, but I just use the tip of a knife.

☐   Take some time this week to review the number of perfumed products in your home. If you can't live without a home fragrance, try a diffuser rather than a candle. And if you can't live without a candle, switch to unscented beeswax.

9 Plastics at home

We urgently need to reduce the quantity of plastic we ingest, and the amount we release into the environment. Ninety-five per cent of adults are believed to have traces of the synthetic chemical bisphenol A (BPA), a hormone disrupter that is found in many plastics, in their bodies. There's no one, clear culprit. We're also continuously exposed to microplastics in our water supply and food chain. As mentioned earlier, research into the impact of microplastics on human health is at an early stage, but it's not looking positive.

Try to reduce the amount of plastic you ingest by:

☐   Eating very little processed food, which will reduce your exposure to the plastic packaging it comes in. Heavily processed and packaged foods absorb chemicals from the plastics they're wrapped in.

☐   Using beeswax wraps instead of clingfilm – they're brilliant!

☐ Decanting food into a glass or china container before
    putting it in the microwave.

☐ Investing in a water filter system for your kitchen.

☐ Carrying a stainless-steel water bottle and coffee
    cup with you.

10 Reduce pesticide exposure

Like pollution, pesticides are impossible to avoid. We're exposed
to multiple toxins via agricultural pesticides, the impact of which
is poorly understood. Government guidelines set clear maximum
residue limits (MRLs) for individual pesticides. These MRLs
are set below the level at which the pesticides could be harmful
to human health. But – *big* but – this doesn't take into account
the cocktail effect caused by multiple pesticides being used on a
single crop. Ninety-two per cent of oranges and 86 per cent of
pears tested in the UK in 2017 contained multiple residues. Over
one-third of each crop contained five or more different residues.
With different pesticides linked to increased risk of heart disease, breast cancer, Alzheimer's and Parkinson's, among other
diseases, we need to do what we can to minimise their impact
as we age.

• Organic produce can reduce this toxic load, but it's not
  always cheap – or available. Pesticide Action Network
  UK produces an annual list of the Clean 15 and the Dirty
  Dozen – the least and most pesticide-ridden produce. It's
  a good indication of where we should put our money if
  we want to buy some organic produce.

- Washing all fruit and veg well does help, but many pesticides are now systemic, meaning they penetrate the whole crop, not just the exterior.
- It's not just fruit and veg that are heavily treated: after researching this issue I've switched to organic rice. Regular rice is also subjected to multiple treatments, with over half the rice available in the UK containing pesticide cocktails.

Pesticide cocktails: the Dirty Dozen and the Clean 15

These lists are produced, and updated annually, by the Pesticide Action Network UK (pan-uk.org). They focus on the produce most and least likely to contain multiple pesticide residues and are based on 2012–2017 data published by the Expert Committee on Pesticide Residues. The percentages are of produce with multiple pesticide residues.

The Dirty Dozen

Grapefruit: 97%
Oranges 96%
Lemons and limes 91%
Strawberries 84%
Pears 84%
Grapes 75%
Cherries 72%
Peaches 72%
Parsnips 69%
Asparagus 66%
Apples 64%
Apricots 64%

The Clean 15

Beetroot 0%
Corn on the cob 0%
Mushrooms 0%
Figs 0%
Rhubarb 0%
Swede 0%
Turnip 0%
Onions 1%
Avocado 2%
Cauliflower 3%
Radish 4%
Sweet potatoes 6%
Broad beans 8%
Leeks 8%
Pumpkin 8%

Don't house plants clean the air, too?

When we started the Age-Well Project, we read multiple
articles about the power of indoor plants to improve air
quality at home. NASA research from the late 1980s[26] found
that when indoor plants convert carbon dioxide to oxygen
via photosynthesis they also scrub the air of potentially
carcinogenic compounds such as formaldehyde and benzene.
The report recommended several plants as effective air
purifiers:

- English ivy
- Spider plant
- Peace lily
- Chinese evergreen
- Bamboo palm

I invested in a collection of these – which looks very pretty – and hoped they were doing their work. More recently, however, researchers have pointed out that the conditions of the NASA study – multiple plants in a small, enclosed space, optimal light for photosynthesis – aren't replicated in a domestic environment. But having plants in the home has been found to reduce stress,[27] improve feelings of well-being and increase energy levels. I find caring for them rather therapeutic, too.

Plan for an age-well life this week

The future, as they say, is what you make it. Up to a point. There are elements that we can't control: a global pandemic, a sudden illness or diagnosis, loss and bereavement, financial issues. But in many instances we can make choices about how we live out the second halves of our lives. We have more freedoms than any generation that has come before us, more opportunities, and – we have to hope – more years to enjoy them.

This section is different from others in the book, as there are more questions than answers, and three broad areas for you to consider: your environment, the world of work and your age-well future. It's easy to bury our heads in the sand and think,

Everything's fine as it is, but sometimes we need to embrace change, step beyond our current vision of ourselves and see other possibilities. The more time and thought we invest in planning our futures, the happier and healthier we will be.

Try this

Take a moment now to visualise how you want life to be as you get older. Imagine you're watching a film of your future life. Where are you? Who are you with? How do you feel? Now take a freeze-frame from the film and examine it. You might be laughing on a beach, walking somewhere beautiful or studying a fascinating painting. You might be running a large company, or just running!

Write down what you see in the freeze-frame. Imagine that you're writing a script for your future life:

Now think about how you can achieve that, even if it is just a small step on the way.

Your age-well environment

The WHO estimates that by 2050 the number of people over the age of 60 will be two billion. By 2019 this age group had already outnumbered children under five. Older citizens are taking over the world, but is the world ready for us?

The towns and cities we live in are unlikely to have been designed with an older population in mind. And what worked for us as young adults, working and possibly raising families, might not be so conducive to ageing well. In 2007 the WHO created a Global Age-Friendly Cities guide which examined eight aspects of urban living worldwide:

- Outdoor spaces and buildings
- Transportation
- Housing
- Social participation
- Respect and social inclusion
- Civic participation and employment
- Communication and information
- Community support and health services

It found, as you can imagine, a vastly mixed bag of experiences for older people across the globe.[28] But the list is a useful lens through which to view your own community (see the checklist over the next few pages). Are you content with the services offered in all these eight sectors in your area? If not, what are you going to do about it?

As the fastest-growing global demographic, we have the power to complain and campaign, to help shape the world the way in which we want to see it as we age. That might be as simple as signing a petition to stop local public loos being closed down (lack of such amenities is a big issue in the WHO report) to joining Friends of the Earth to protest against pollution to campaigning for public office yourself. All these would make the world a better place. And, of course, getting involved reaps benefits in terms of socialisation and the feel-good factor of volunteering.

What are you waiting for? None of us is ageing in a vacuum: we have to make it work for everyone.

How does your locality measure up?

Rate your locality according to the WHO age-friendly cities guide. Grade each issue out of 10, and scribble down any notes or areas you want to research further.

What does your local area offer by way of outdoor spaces, leisure facilities and public buildings?

Mark out of 10:

Are you happy with public transport links in your area? Would you be able to get around if you couldn't drive?

Mark out of 10:

Does your current home lend itself to ageing – how accessible is it? Would it be too big to manage if you were incapacitated in some way?

Mark out of 10:

Are there activities and organisations nearby that you would like to get involved with?

Mark out of 10:

Do you think older people are valued, considered and included?

Mark out of 10:

Are there opportunities for you to get involved locally, and continue to work if you would like to?

Mark out of 10:

Is it easy to find information about what's available in your area?

Mark out of 10:

How accessible are health services and other forms of care that you might need as you get older, such as social care, and so on?

Mark out of 10:

Ageing well and the world of work

Many of the world's SuperAgers keep working long after they could have collected their gold clock and retired. A long and idle retirement might seem appealing, but the evidence suggests that the grit and determination required to keep us in the workplace is more beneficial to our long-term health. Some of the SuperAgers we met for *The Age-Well Project* were still working into their nineties. That is pretty extreme, of course, but some form of work – it could be voluntary or part-time – confers huge health benefits. In her book *Extra Time: 10 Lessons for an Ageing World*, Camilla Cavendish asks the question, 'What if retirement makes you old?' She advocates 'unretiring' and going back to work, or retiring *to* something.

Work doesn't have to mean slogging away in a windowless office. For older Okinawans, it means tending their gardens, cooking and looking after their grandchildren. For those with an enduring love of art, whatever its form, it means painting, writing, composing, singing, sculpting or dancing. What does it mean for you?

Recent research found that just eight hours of paid work a week boosted mental health and life satisfaction.[29] It also boosts the bank balance, of course, gives us purpose and allows for inter-generational contact (which has been found to reduce ageism towards older adults).

How to age well at work

- Does your workplace have a policy to prevent age discrimination? Be aware of what it says and who to talk to if you experience discrimination.
- If you're finding your job stressful or tough, can you afford to go part-time? Could you work from home one day a week to ease the burden of commuting? Or could you

work more flexible hours to avoid the rush-hour crush?

- A government survey found that older people are less likely than younger workers to receive workplace training. If you feel you could benefit from new skills, ask for training.
- Keep learning – 40 per cent of 55–64-year-olds have undertaken no formal training or education since leaving school. Don't let your skills lag behind.
- Age well during your working day – get daylight on your way into work, stretch at your desk, walk at lunchtime and enjoy the mental stimulation that employment brings.
- As we know from Week 3, sitting for too long creates myriad health problems: find ways to break up long sedentary periods at your desk, even if it's offering to make your colleagues a cup of tea!

Your age-well future

Assuming that you're in good health as you get older, where is it going to take you? The last six weeks have all been about having a plan for the present. Now it's time to plan for the future.

What does your age-well future look like? Where will you live, with whom and how will you pay for it? There are many questions we need to ask ourselves if we want to age well in every aspect of our lives.

Give your life an age-well MOT

Rate the following areas of your life out of 10, and mark down what you could do to improve your score if you need to.

Money Review your finances with forward planning in mind. How's your pension looking?

Mark out of 10:

Environment Does the place you live in now give you opportunities to age well? Are there green spaces and a sense of community? How did it match up to the WHO age-friendly cities criteria when you worked through the list on pages 224–225?

Mark out of 10:

Work Do you want to continue working, or retire, or retrain? How do you see your future in the world of work?

Mark out of 10:

Education Could you learn new skills that would help you in your current job, get you back to work or enable you to make the most of retirement? Does your current skill set suit your goals?

Mark out of 10:

Relationships Evaluate your relationships. Which of them will bolster you as you strive to age well – and which need work?

Mark out of 10:

Your age-well goals Discuss how you're going to age well with the people around you: partners, children, friends. Do you share the same goals?

Mark out of 10:

Activities Think about the hobbies and activities you're taking into the future with you. Do they stimulate and challenge you?

Mark out of 10:

Mindset How do you feel about ageing? A positive frame of mind is the most useful tool you have as you go forward from here.

Mark out of 10:

Your personal age-well plan – how to live

Review what you've achieved this week: how have you changed your environment? What's worked? What hasn't? What's been hardest? What's been easiest? How do you feel about your age-well future?

I've listed the key actions again here to remind you. Tick the points that you're going to consider in the future. There's a line for notes and reminders too.

☐   Reduce your car usage and walk more.

☐   Rethink the cleaning products you use in your home.

☐   Switch to less harsh alternatives for cleaning if necessary.

☐   Review your skincare products.

☐   Consider the number of scented products in your home.

☐   Cut down on the amount of plastic you use.

☐ Avoid pesticide exposure.

☐ Rate how age-friendly your locality is.

☐ Consider the role of work in your life as you age.

☐ How was your age-well MOT? Which areas of your life need more work?

Set your intentions for the future: how will you live from now on?

Based on the tick list you've just created, write out your 'how to live' intentions for your own age-well plan; for example, *I will rethink my cleaning products, reduce my plastics and review my future plans with my family*. These and your other intentions will create a list of good age-well habits that will last a lifetime.

Refer back to your age-well goals, personalised health plan and age-well eating, moving, sleeping and 'being' plans from the last five weeks. Have you been able to keep to your age-well plan this week? Write out your age-well purpose again here to help you remember it:

PROFESSOR CAROL BRAYNE, CAMBRIDGE INSTITUTE OF PUBLIC HEALTH

'Help the world to age well'

Cambridge University professor Carol Brayne, CBE, is Professor of Public Health Medicine and Director of the Cambridge Institute of Public Health. She looks very broadly at the issues around dementia, dementia care and how, as a society, we can best cope with rising numbers of older people with multiple health problems.

As a public-health expert, Professor Brayne emphasises the role of society, not just the individual, in healthy living: 'We need to lobby for the changes that make societies healthy, which make environments healthy, so that it becomes easy for people to exercise, easy for people to eat healthily. It's a much bigger thing than just suggesting that people change their behaviour – we need to change the way we organise our societies. For example, fast-food outlets are targeted into socio-economically deprived areas, so those companies that provide the profits for our economic system and our pension funds are targeting the poor with fast food, which is damaging their brains for later life.'

She's clear that poor health shouldn't be seen as an individual failure to follow guidelines: 'There's this idea of blame, and it's aimed at people who live in more deprived areas. There's a danger that this will lead to people thinking: *You've got all the information and you carried on smoking, so you should pay for your care*. But that punitive approach is misguided. We can't create a society in which that can happen and then blame the individual for the choice they made – it's not fair.'

Carol does look after her own health, and, at 61, is slim and fit. Exercise has always been very important to her – she cycles, swims and hikes – but, again, she emphasises the role of society in keeping us all fit: 'I think it's really important that we create environments in which it is pleasant for everybody to get outside. There need to be paths and places to go. They need to be safe, too, and engage all generations.' And engagement goes beyond physical activity: 'In later life, social engagement is really important, too – in general people recover better from cognitive impairment if they are socially engaged.'

As we're talking, she tasks me to imagine a redesigned supermarket that would engage shoppers both physically and mentally. The car park would be a short walk away from the shop, not right next to it, and we'd have to navigate a cobbled path to the entrance. Cobbles work on our balance,

'We need to challenge our balance systems so that we don't let our bodies atrophy,' she explains. And when we get inside, a shop worker would greet us, so we'd benefit from social engagement, too. These are simple changes, but ones Carol believes could make a huge difference to our health: 'We need to find ways to help the people who find it difficult. I hate to use the word "nudge", but it's about making it possible, and then often there is a positive reinforcement cycle.'

The most important thing we can do, however, is to engage with good health as a society-wide issue, not just an individual one. She urges us all to get involved: 'I'd really love to be able to create a social movement for ageing well – it ought to be everybody's right.'

CONCLUSION

Over to You

Congratulations! You now have a personal age-well plan, with a list of to-dos that you can work into daily life and refer back to in the years to come. Take some time now to look back over the last six weeks and think about what's worked best for you, what you've enjoyed and what you still need to work on. Maybe there's something you *didn't* enjoy but which you know is important. Review the personal age-well plan you created at the end of each chapter to remind yourself of how far you've come and the fundamentals: eating more vegetables, exercising, prioritising sleep, having fun connecting to people and planning your future.

From six weeks' planning to the rest of your life

Rate your transformation. How do you feel? What do you still want to work on? Write it down here:

A final thought

The ageing process is rarely perfect, with many bumps in the road ahead. But the commitment to create an age-well life is empowering. In a world designed to make us sick, fat and old, reclaiming our health by taking positive steps to age well is a radical and powerful act, so keep working on your age-well plan every day and every week and you will reap the benefits in the coming years.

An age-well life is about breathing the fresh air, eating the chocolate, calling the long-lost friend. It's about stepping away from the harshness of modern life: stretching at our desks – not being chained to them; walking in the woods – not sitting in the car; bed and a book – not being glued to a screen; cooking whole food – not microwaving a ready meal. I urge you to continue to challenge yourself, each day and each week, to age well.

Stay with the age-well community. Join us on:

- Facebook: @theagewellproject and @susanasaundershealth
- Instagram: @agewellproject and @susanasaundershealth
- Twitter: @age_wellproject
- Websites: agewellproject.com and susansaundershealth.com

There's lots of support, advice and all-round cheerleading available as we all age well together.

Bon chance on your journey – make it a good one.

APPENDIX I

Know Your Numbers

The figures below are general guidelines. I urge you to check the websites listed and talk to a health professional. Getting to grips with test results means we're better able to take control of our health.

Body Mass Index*

Less than 19	Underweight
19–24.9	Healthy weight
25–29.9	Overweight
30–34.9	Obese
35 or higher	Morbidly obese

Blood pressure*

If your blood pressure is above 120/80, you should take steps to bring it down. Although that's not technically in the 'high' range, it can cause health problems. bloodpressureuk.org has lots of advice.

*Source: www.nhs.uk

Systolic blood pressure

Less than 90	Low	
90–119	Good	
120–139	Normal/ pre-hypertensive	Below 120 is ideal
140–159	High	Above 130 is considered high for diabetes patients
160 or higher	Very high	

Diastolic blood pressure

Less than 60	Low	
60–79	Good	
80–89	Normal	Below 80 is ideal
90–99	High	
100 or higher	Very high	

Total cholesterol

Use your total cholesterol as a general indicator; a full lipid profile will measure the proportion of LDL (aka 'bad' cholesterol) to HDL (aka 'good' cholesterol) as well as triglycerides. Talk to your doctor about the proportions revealed by your test. In the UK, your results will be given to you in mmol/L (millimoles per litre). www.heartuk.org.uk has information about interpreting your cholesterol check results and what to do with them.

Less than 5.0	Good level
5.0–6.49	Raised level
6.5 or higher	High level

Blood glucose levels

The figures given below are the normal ranges for people without diabetes. They are given in mmol/L. Blood glucose levels vary according to whether or not you are in a fasted state when you take the test.

| When fasting | 4.0–5.4 mmol/L |
| Two hours after eating | Up to 7.8 mmol/L |

www.diabetes.org.uk has more information about blood glucose tests.

APPENDIX II

Full Pantry List

Here is a complete list of the items that I keep in my kitchen to help me knock up age-well meals and snacks. It's taken me years to build up to this and I have a lot of mouths to feed. Please don't feel you have to rush out and buy all this at once.

Larder

A wide variety of nuts, seeds and dried fruit, but always Brazil nuts, cashew nuts, walnuts and pumpkin seeds.

Almond butter
Brown rice
Buckwheat groats
Cacao nibs
Chia seeds
Dark chocolate (at least 70 per cent cocoa solids)
Date syrup
Flours: whole wheat, spelt, chickpea, buckwheat
Freekeh
Hemp hearts (shelled hemp seeds)
Lentils: red, black, brown, Puy, cooked (in pouches)
Maple syrup
Medjool dates
Mung dhal or split peas plus other beans and pulses that need soaking and cooking

Nutritional yeast

Oats – jumbo and porridge

Passata and tinned tomatoes

Peanut butter

Pomegranate molasses

Quinoa

Raw cacao powder

Raw honey

Tins of cooked beans –
chickpeas, butterbeans,
black beans, kidney beans,
cannellini beans

Tins of sardines and tuna

Wholewheat couscous

Wholewheat pasta
and noodles

Avocados

Bananas, apples and seasonal
fruit

Lemons and limes

Onions and garlic

Sweet potatoes and carrots

Black tea

Coffee

Green tea (loose leaf)

Herbal teas – camomile,
lavender, tulsi, nettle

Dried herbs and blends: bay
leaves, bouquet garni,
oregano, za'atar

Spices and blends: allspice,
baharat, berbere, black

pepper, chilli, cinnamon,
cloves, cumin, fennel seeds,
mixed spice, paprika, ras-
el-hanout, sumac, sweet
smoked paprika, turmeric

Apple cider vinegar

Coconut oil (raw, extra virgin)

Extra-virgin olive oil

Olive oil

Red wine vinegar

Rice bran oil

Sesame oil

Walnut oil (or avocado)

Fridge

Anchovies

Butter

Capers

Eggs

Feta cheese

Ginger (in a jar or fresh root ginger)

Ground flax seeds

Hummus

Kefir

Miso paste – red and white

Mustard

Parmesan cheese

Plain live yogurt

Seasonal brassica vegetables – broccoli, kale, sprouts, cauliflower

Seasonal leafy green vegetables – spinach, cavolo nero

Soft herbs – coriander, basil, flat-leaf parsley, mint

Tahini

Tofu

Freezer

Avocado

Banana slices

Blueberries

Chicken livers

Chopped spinach

Corn

Edamame beans

Leftover cooked grains and pulses

Salmon roe

Tempeh

Wild salmon fillets

Miscellaneous

Beeswax wraps (to reduce waste and the amount of plastic that comes into contact with food)

Water filter

APPENDIX III

Menu Plan and Recipes

This plan gives you a week's worth of breakfasts, lunches and dinners to follow while you're working through Week 2: How to Eat. It's a lot to prep and cook, I know. But even if you grab lunch at work, eat out or batch-cook during the week – anything to make life easier – use this plan to give you inspiration and guidance. As long as you stick to my berries–greens–greens mantra, add some beans and work on your intermittent-fasting window, you'll be taking giant strides towards eating to age well.

A note on portions: almost all the recipes can be scaled up or down, depending on the number of people you're feeding. With teenagers in the house, we tend to make our own breakfasts and lunches and come together for dinner, which is why day-time meals are for one or two, and evening meals are for four. I wanted to give you a sense of how I've evolved my cooking and eating at home to help me age well, while still fitting in the demands of family life.

A note on meat: the meal plan contains very little meat – just some roast chicken and chicken livers. I've kept the meat intake to a minimum this week as I'd like to encourage you to experiment with vegetables and pulses as much as possible. I do believe meat has a role to play in a healthy age-well diet, however, and I love roast lamb on a Sunday or a treat-night steak and chips occasionally. If you do too, please continue to enjoy them!

A shopping list for the week's menu can be found at agewellproject.com

Day 1 – Sunday

Sunday might not be the obvious day to start a one-week plan, but I use the day to get ahead with meal prep. During the week, the time between getting home from work and getting dinner on the table is scant, so the more prepared I am, the better. I cook a Sunday roast so that I can use the leftovers for dinner on Monday, and I make a bean dish in advance to eat on Tuesday. If I can add a few snacks and breakfasts to that too, I feel I'm winning at life before the week's even begun!

Brunch: The Age-Well Fry-Up

I tend to eat only two meals on a Sunday: a big brunch-style meal and an early evening roast. This gives me an opportunity to extend my fasting time, and to get in some exercise or a long walk on Sunday morning while I'm in a fasted state. It also means I can indulge in afternoon snacks and treats to keep me going, if required!

Serves 2
1 tbsp olive oil
100g mushrooms, sliced
2 large handfuls of spinach

2–4 large eggs, depending on appetite

2 slices of wholegrain bread

100g smoked salmon

2 tbsp kimchi or sauerkraut

½ avocado (optional), sliced

salt and ground black pepper

1 Heat the oil in a large frying pan over a medium/high heat and add the mushrooms. Cook for 5 minutes or until they have released their liquid and it starts to reduce, then add the spinach. Season well and let the spinach wilt. Tip into a heatproof dish and keep warm.

2 Put a large saucepan of water on to boil (or two saucepans if you're cooking 4 eggs), and crack the eggs into separate small bowls (they poach better when you don't crack them straight into the water, for some reason). Once the water in the saucepan/s has come to a rolling boil, slip the eggs into the water. Wait for the water to come back to the boil then set a timer for 2 minutes 15 seconds.

3 Meanwhile, toast the bread, layer the smoked salmon on top of it and put onto each plate with the mushrooms and spinach. As soon as the eggs are ready, scoop them out of the water and top your fry-up with the eggs, then add the kimchi and avocado, if using.

Dinner: Roast Chicken

Beans and vegetables cook alongside this slow-roast chicken, so – with the addition of some greens – you have a complete meal. A dollop of the Punchy Herb Sauce takes it to the next level, though. Keep leftover meat for tomorrow night's dinner.

Serves 4, plus leftovers

1 tbsp finely chopped rosemary

1 tsp dried oregano

1 tsp sweet smoked paprika

1 tsp salt

2 tbsp olive oil

1 large chicken, preferably free-range and organic

1 lemon, halved

2 carrots, chopped into rough chunks

3 leeks, cut into rough chunks

6 garlic cloves, peeled

2 × 400g cans cannellini or flageolet beans, drained and rinsed

½ bottle of dry white wine

salt and ground black pepper

green vegetables and Punchy Herb Sauce (see page 271)
    (optional), to serve

1 Preheat the oven to 150°C/300°F/Gas 2. Put the rosemary in a small bowl and add the oregano, paprika, salt and oil. Add several grinds of black pepper and mix well. Put the chicken in an ovenproof dish, ideally one with a lid. Rub the herb mix over the chicken and pop the lemon halves up its bum.

2 Arrange the carrots, leeks and garlic around the chicken, pour over the wine and season lightly with salt and pepper. Cover tightly with the lid or use foil and roast for 1 hour.

3 Carefully remove the lid (or peel back the foil) – watch out for hot steam – and add the beans. There should be plenty of liquid, but if it looks a little dry, add a splash of water. Replace the lid/foil and return to the oven for 1 hour.

4 Remove the lid and cook for 15 minutes so that the chicken can brown. Take out of the oven and allow to rest while you

cook your green veg. Carve the chicken and, using tongs, squeeze a little juice from the lemon halves in the cavity into the bean mixture. Taste for seasoning then ladle into shallow bowls with the chicken slices on top and the greens alongside. Add the herb sauce if you like.

Prepare for tomorrow

After dinner, strip the chicken meat from the carcass and put it on a plate in the fridge. Throw the bones into a large saucepan with a roughly chopped onion, a couple of chopped carrots (no need to peel them), a stalk of lemongrass, a 2cm chunk of peeled ginger, 3 star anise, 1 cinnamon stick, 1 tsp coriander seeds, 1 tsp Chinese five-spice powder and 1 tsp peppercorns. Cover with cold water, bring to the boil, then reduce the heat and simmer for 2 hours, or 3 hours, if you have time. This stock forms the basis of tomorrow night's Chicken Pho (page 249).

I also like to prep the Black Bean Chilli for Tuesday (page 252), if I have time.

Before I go to bed, I prep my breakfast mix for the next couple of days. Put 2 tbsp chia seeds, 4 tbsp oats and 2 tsp ground cinnamon in a bowl. Mix and add milk (any type, I like oat) or water to cover. This is enough for two portions. Leave in the fridge overnight.

You could also bake the Spiced Tahini Granola (see page 257), if you want to get ahead.

Day 2 – Monday

Breakfast: Classic Breakfast Pot

This is what I eat for my (mid-morning) breakfast day in and day out. It's always slightly different, depending on the combination of berries, spices and toppings that I use. You'll need half the breakfast mix you made last night.

Serves 1

1 portion (½ quantity) breakfast mix (page 247)

50g berries, fresh or frozen (blueberries, plus what's in season or in the freezer)

½ tsp ground mixed spice

2 tbsp kefir or natural live yogurt

2 tsp nut butter

toppings of your choice, such as chopped nuts, bee pollen, banana slices

Dollop the breakfast mix into a bowl, or portable container if you're taking this to work. Stir in the berries, spice and kefir. Drizzle over the nut butter and add toppings of your choice.

Lunch: Sardines on Toast

Serves 1

Beans, greens and sardines form the backbone of my age-well lunches at home, often with a small slice of wholegrain bread.

The simplest lunch of all is a small tin of sardines (the cheap ones, with bones) mashed onto a slice of buttered toast, with a side of greens. I sauté kale, spinach, chard or broccoli – anything

I have – in 1 tbsp olive oil, season well and squeeze over a little lemon. I pile this up alongside my sardine toast.

Then it's back to my desk with a cup of green tea, a couple of squares of very dark chocolate, three Brazil nuts (for selenium) and a few dried cherries or fresh berries, depending on the time of year.

Dinner: Leftover Chicken Pho

This meal is very much a blueprint. If you don't have leftover chicken to hand, or if you don't eat meat, it works just as well with vegetable stock and tofu cubes (see vegetarian version below). It's a flavoursome vehicle for plenty of vegetables and very adaptable.

Serves 4
1½ litres chicken stock, strained, from last night's meal prep
1 tbsp fish sauce, plus extra to serve
1 tbsp lime juice
2 heads of pak choi, shredded
100g mushrooms, sliced
300g wholegrain rice noodles
leftover chicken, chopped

Toppings:
2 carrots, grated
4 spring onions, finely sliced
2 large handfuls of bean sprouts
4 tbsp chopped fresh coriander
4 tbsp chopped fresh mint leaves
4 tbsp crushed roasted peanuts

1 lime, cut into four wedges
1 red chilli, deseeded and finely sliced

1 Heat the chicken stock and add the fish sauce, lime juice and vegetables. Cook the noodles in a separate pan for 2 minutes or until just tender, or according to the packet instructions.
2 When the vegetables are almost cooked, add the chicken meat and make sure it's thoroughly heated through.
3 Put the various toppings in individual bowls or a large plate on the table so that people can help themselves. Divide the noodles between four bowls and ladle over the broth, vegetables and chicken. Allow people to add their own toppings to make the pho their own.

Vegetarian version

If you're making this from scratch, fry 1 chopped onion (or 2 shallots) and 2 garlic cloves in a little oil over a medium heat for 6 minutes or until caramelised and golden. Add 1½ litres vegetable stock, a stalk of lemongrass, a 2cm chunk of peeled ginger, 3 star anise, 1 cinnamon stick, 1 tsp coriander seeds, 1 tsp Chinese five-spice powder and 1 tsp peppercorns. Bring to the boil, then reduce the heat and simmer for 15 minutes, then strain. Add the fish sauce (or use soy sauce as a vegetarian equivalent), lime juice and vegetables. Continue with the recipe as above. Replace the chicken with 300g of cubed tofu.

Day 3 – Tuesday

Breakfast: Black Forest Gateau Pot

I try to avoid so-called superfoods and focus on readily available, everyday age-well foods, but I do make an exception for cacao. The word refers to the raw cocoa bean before it's processed to make chocolate. It delivers a chocolatey taste and is packed with powerful antioxidants but without the sugar and fat that come with refined chocolate. For this breakfast, you'll need the remaining half of the breakfast mix you made on Sunday.

Serves 1
1 portion (½ quantity) breakfast pot mix (page 247)
milk, if needed
1 tbsp raw cacao powder
50g fresh or defrosted frozen cherries
2 tbsp live natural yogurt
1 tbsp raw cacao nibs

If the breakfast pot mix has got a little stiff overnight, loosen with some extra milk. Stir in the cacao powder and cherries. Top with yogurt and cacao nibs.

Lunch: Beans and Greens on Toast

Serves 1
Time for another 'something on toast' if I'm working at home. I sauté a chopped leek in 1 tbsp olive oil, add a few mushrooms if I have them, a couple of large handfuls of greens and 2 tbsp of rinsed tinned beans. I season them with salt, pepper and a

squeeze of lemon before piling the mixture onto a piece of toast.

A quick rummage in the fridge usually produces something to top it all off – a crumble of feta cheese, a drizzle of tahini, some Quick Pickled Red Onion (see page 262), toasted nuts or seeds, or a dollop of Punchy Herb Sauce (page 271).

Dinner: Black Bean Chilli and Sweet Potato Tacos

I try to make this black bean chilli on a Sunday so that I'm halfway to a meal on Tuesday night. Sweet potatoes are terrific age-well foods: high in fibre and the antioxidant beta-carotene. They are popular with the long-lived Blue Zone residents of Okinawa and the Nicoya Peninsula.

Serves 4
1 tbsp olive oil
1 onion, chopped
2 garlic cloves, finely chopped
1 tsp dried oregano
1 tbsp ground cumin
1 tsp ground cinnamon
2 tsp sweet smoked paprika
½ tsp chilli powder, or to taste
½ tsp ground turmeric
2 × 400g tins black beans, one drained and rinsed, one not
200g tin or carton tomato passata
salt and ground black pepper

For the sweet potatoes:
2 tsp ground cumin
1 tsp ground cinnamon

1 tsp sweet smoked paprika

1 tsp salt

1 tsp chilli powder, or to taste

2 tbsp olive oil

3 sweet potatoes, cut into cubes

To serve:

8 taco shells or 4 large wholewheat wraps

4 lime wedges

avocado slices

chopped lettuce

tomato salsa

1 Preheat the oven to 180°C/350°F/Gas 4. Start with the sweet potatoes: mix the spices with the oil in a large bowl then add the sweet potato cubes. Mix to make sure the cubes are well coated. Spread them out onto a baking tray and roast for 30–40 minutes until crispy and starting to brown on the outside and soft on the inside.

2 If you haven't made the chilli already, crack on with it while the sweet potatoes are roasting. Heat the 1 tbsp of the oil in a saucepan over a medium heat and cook the onion for 5 minutes. Add the garlic, oregano and spices. Cook for 30 seconds, adding a splash of water if the spices are in danger of burning.

3 Add the beans, including the cooking liquid from one tin, and the passata. Bring to the boil then reduce the heat and simmer for 20 minutes, stirring occasionally, until the mixture has thickened. Taste and season well with salt and pepper.

4 Fill tacos or wraps with the chilli and sweet potatoes, then squeeze over some lime and let everyone help themselves to avocado, lettuce and salsa.

Day 4 – Wednesday

Breakfast: Sweet Green Smoothie

I know green smoothies are a bit of a 'wellness' cliché, but look past that to the opportunity to start the day with a big portion of greens. They're so simple to make if you have a powerful blender or food processor. I use a Nutribullet.

> *Serves 1*
> 1 small handful of kale, chopped
> 1 large handful of baby spinach
> a chunk of cucumber
> ½ ripe banana
> 4 cubes of frozen mango
> 1 tsp ginger pulp from a jar, or 1cm fresh ginger, peeled
>   and grated
> juice of 1 lime
> 1 tbsp hemp hearts or nut butter
> 100ml milk (any type) or water
> 1 tsp matcha (Japanese green tea powder) (optional)

Put all the ingredients in a blender or food processor and whizz until completely smooth. Drink immediately or seal well and take to work to break your fast mid-morning.

Lunch: Brain-Boosting Salmon Salad with Kefir and Horseradish Dressing

This simple salad makes use of wild tinned salmon, which is not a very fashionable ingredient, but it is packed with brain-boosting omega-3 fatty acids DHA and EPA. If you can get hold of a jar of salmon roe and can cope with the taste (and the price), a teaspoon or two make a great addition to this dish.

Serves 1

2 large handfuls of rocket leaves (or a mix of rocket and
    watercress)

100g tinned wild salmon

60g tinned chickpeas (about a quarter of a can), drained
    and rinsed

½ ripe avocado (optional), chopped

1–2 tsp wild salmon roe, to taste (optional)

For the dressing:

4 tbsp kefir

2 tsp horseradish sauce, or to taste (every brand seems to vary
    wildly in potency)

2 tsp lemon juice

2 tsp wholegrain mustard

1 tsp finely chopped dill (optional)

salt and ground black pepper

1 Put all the dressing ingredients in a bowl and mix well.

2 Spread the salad leaves out on a plate and layer on the salmon, chickpeas and avocado, if using. Drizzle over the dressing – you'll have some spare for another day. Top with the salmon roe, if using.

Dinner: Tempeh and Miso Stir-Fry

I'm an enormous fan of tempeh – this age-well superfood deserves a wider audience. It's an Indonesian food, made of fermented soya beans, which have been pressed into a block. Unlike its Japanese cousin, tofu, it's made from the whole bean, so it's high in fibre. Find it in health-food shops or online.

Serves 4
300g brown rice
2 tbsp olive, sesame or rapeseed oil
1 tbsp low-salt soy sauce
200g tempeh, cut into 1cm cubes
2 garlic cloves, finely chopped
1 tsp ginger pulp from a jar, or 1cm fresh ginger, peeled
    and grated
2 red peppers, deseeded and cut into strips
1 head of broccoli, cut into florets
200g mushrooms, sliced

For the sauce:
1½ tbsp dark miso
2 tbsp mirin (Japanese rice wine)
2 tbsp rice vinegar (or cider vinegar)
2 tbsp tahini

1 Put the brown rice in a large saucepan with double the volume of water. Bring it to the boil then cover it, reduce the heat and simmer for 20 minutes. Remove from the heat and leave, covered, for 5–10 minutes until the water is absorbed and the grains are tender. (Or follow the packet instructions.)

2 Meanwhile, put the sauce ingredients in a bowl and whisk together, adding a little water to get a smooth paste, the consistency of double cream. Set aside.

3 Heat 1 tbsp of the oil in a wok or large frying pan over a high heat. Add the soy sauce and tempeh cubes, and fry until they absorb the soy sauce and start to form a crust. When they are browned, tip them out of the pan and put to one side.

4 Add the remaining oil to the pan and heat. Stir-fry the garlic and ginger for 30 seconds, then add the vegetables. Toss them in the pan until they start to soften. Add 2 tbsp water and cover with a lid. Cook for 2 minutes.

5 Return the tempeh to the pan, then stir-fry it all together until piping hot. Switch off the heat and drizzle over the sauce (this ensures that the live cultures in the miso aren't destroyed). Serve immediately with the rice.

Day 5 – Thursday

Breakfast: Spiced Tahini Granola

I'm not suggesting that you must find the time to bake granola on a weekday morning, but if you have the opportunity, please do, as this is delicious slightly warm from the oven. As Wednesday night's dinner was a quick stir-fry, you might have been able to carve out a few minutes to prep for today's breakfast. Or this could be part of your Sunday prep. The granola keeps well in an airtight container. I sprinkle 2–3 tablespoons over yogurt or kefir and add lots of berries for a speedy breakfast.

Makes about 8 portions

150g jumbo oats

100g walnuts, crumbled

100g mixed nuts and seeds (such as almonds, Brazil nuts,
     pumpkin seeds), chopped

3 tbsp coconut oil

3 tbsp maple syrup

4 tbsp tahini

2 tsp ground cinnamon

½ tsp ground mixed spice

¼ tsp freshly grated cloves (careful, it's strong stuff, but
     packed with antioxidants)

75g dried fruit, chopped (optional – I prefer it without)

1 Preheat the oven to 150°C/300°F/Gas 2 and line a large
  baking tray with baking parchment. Mix the oats, nuts and
  seeds in a large bowl. Melt the coconut oil, then stir in the
  maple syrup, tahini and spices until well mixed.

2 Pour this over the oat mixture and stir well, ensuring that
  it's all coated with the syrup mix. Empty the mixture onto
  the prepared baking tray and lightly tamp it down so that it
  clumps together.

3 Bake for 15 minutes, then check to ensure it's not burning. Stir
  and return to the oven for another 5–10 minutes until brown
  and crunchy to your taste – but make sure it doesn't burn!
  Remove from the oven and stir in the fruit, if using.

4 Sprinkle a few tablespoons over yogurt or kefir and top
  with berries.

Lunch: Chicken Liver and Pomegranate Salad

Chicken livers, and all offal (organ meats), are a rich source of B vitamins, such as folate and B12, as well as iron, zinc and the fat-soluble vitamins A, D, E and K. They also provide plenty of protein. Try to buy organic if you can.

Serves 2
400g chicken livers
2 tbsp olive oil
2 cloves garlic, finely sliced
2 tbsp pomegranate molasses
Baby leaf spinach and good bread, to serve
2 tbsp pomegranate seeds

1 Rinse the chicken livers in a sieve and snip out any sinew and green-tinged bits.
2 Heat the oil in a large frying pan. Add the livers and season well with salt and pepper. Cook for 6–7 minutes on a medium heat, stirring occasionally. Push them to one side of the pan and add the garlic. Cook for around 30 seconds.
3 Turn the heat right down and add the pomegranate molasses. Stir well and cook for another minute, or until the molasses starts to bubble.
4 Arrange the spinach leaves on two plates and divide the liver mixture between them. Sprinkle over the pomegranate seeds and eat with bread to mop up the juices.

Dinner: Thai Green Smoothie Curry

Edamame beans are unprocessed soya beans that you can buy frozen. They're rich in spermidine, which helps to stimulate autophagy in the body. The sauce for this curry is whizzed up in the blender or Nutribullet to make it smooth and creamy and can be made a little in advance, if you like.

Serves 4
1 tbsp olive oil
2 onions, roughly chopped
2 garlic cloves, finely chopped
2 tsp ginger pulp from a jar, or 2cm fresh ginger, peeled
   and grated
1 tbsp Thai green curry paste (from a jar)
4 big handfuls of chopped kale
4 (about 100g) frozen spinach nuggets, defrosted
a bunch of fresh coriander
400g tin of coconut milk
juice of 1 lime
2 tbsp fish sauce
1 tsp sugar
75g cashew nuts
150g edamame beans
2 courgettes, cubed
brown rice, to serve

1 Heat the oil in a large saucepan over a medium heat and cook the onions, garlic, ginger and Thai curry paste for 5 minutes or until the onion is translucent.
2 Wilt down one big handful of kale in the pan, then add the

spinach, half the bunch of coriander (stalks and all) and the coconut milk. Mix well then tip into a blender or food processor. Add the lime juice, fish sauce and sugar, then blend until smooth. The recipe can be prepped in advance up to here.

3 Put the cashew nuts in a dry pan and toast over a medium-high heat, tossing regularly, for 2–3 minutes or until golden brown. Set aside.

4 Pour the smoothie into a saucepan and heat gently. Add the edamame beans, courgettes and remaining kale, and cook through.

5 Chop the remaining coriander. Serve the curry, topped with the cashew nuts and chopped coriander, with brown rice.

Day 6 – Friday

Breakfast: Savoury Green Smoothie

I know the idea of a savoury green smoothie sounds weird, especially for breakfast, but trust me on this one. It takes a little getting used to, but think of it as a green Virgin Mary and you'll understand how to season it.

Serves 1
large handful of spinach
small handful of kale
chunk of cucumber or ½ courgette
small bunch of parsley (about 15g)
¼ ripe avocado
6 almonds or 1 tbsp almond butter
1 tsp Worcestershire sauce

a few drops of Tabasco sauce or chilli sauce
juice of ½ lemon
salt and ground black pepper

Blend all the ingredients together in a blender or food processor and season with salt and pepper. Serve very cold.

Lunch: Lentil, Feta and Chickpea Salad with Quick Pickled Red Onion

This is a handy and delicious store-cupboard salad. It keeps well in the fridge, too.

Serves 2
2 tbsp walnuts
400g tin of chickpeas, rinsed and drained
250g cooked Puy lentils, from a packet
2 tbsp chopped fresh herbs (such as parsley, basil, coriander)
50g feta cheese

Quick pickled red onion:
1 tsp salt
1 tsp sugar
6 tbsp red wine vinegar
1 red onion, finely sliced into half moons

Dressing:
1 garlic clove, finely chopped
pinch of salt
1 tsp ras-el-hanout spice mix
juice of ½ lemon

2 tbsp tahini

2 tbsp olive oil

2–3 tbsp hot water

1 Start with the pickled red onion. Put the salt in a bowl, and add the sugar and vinegar, then stir well. Add the onion, stir well, then put to one side to macerate.

2 To make the dressing, put the garlic in a small bowl, add the salt, then mash it to a paste (the salt acts as an abrasive). Mix together all the remaining ingredients, except the hot water. Use sufficient water to thin the dressing until it's the consistency of double cream.

3 Toast the walnuts in a small dry frying pan over a medium heat. Set aside. Mix the chickpeas, lentils and herbs in a serving bowl. Drizzle over dressing and top with the feta and walnuts. Drain the onions and add some to the bowl, to taste. (You'll have onions left over, but they go with everything.)

Dinner: Green Dhal

Friday night is curry night!

Serves 4

2 tbsp coconut oil

2 onions, chopped

2 garlic cloves, finely chopped

1 tsp ginger pulp from a jar, or 1 cm fresh ginger, peeled
    and grated

1 tsp ground turmeric

2 tsp garam masala (see Tip)

250g mung dhal or red lentils

100g (about 4 nuggets) frozen chopped spinach

½–1 tsp salt, to taste

juice of ½ lemon

2 tbsp fresh chopped coriander

Greek yogurt, mango chutney and 4 wholewheat
 chapattis, to serve

1 Heat 1 tbsp of the oil in a large saucepan over a medium heat and cook 1 onion until soft. Add the garlic, ginger, turmeric and 1 tsp of the garam masala. Cook for 1 minute more, then stir in the mung dhal or lentils. Add 1 litre of water and bring to the boil. Reduce the heat and simmer for 20–30 minutes until the pulses have collapsed and you have a thick, soup-like consistency.

2 Stir in the frozen spinach and let it wilt in the dhal. Stir frequently so that the mix doesn't stick to the base of the pan. Add the salt to taste and the lemon juice.

3 Meanwhile, fry the remaining onion in the remaining oil over a medium heat for 7 minutes or until starting to crisp, then add the remaining garam masala.

4 Stir in 1 tbsp of the coriander. Serve topped with the fried onion mix and the remaining coriander. Dollop on yogurt and mango chutney, then serve with chapattis.

Tip I cook this dish a lot, so I've invested in a Bart garam masala mill, which I love. It delivers freshly ground spices every time, which makes a big difference to the finished dish.

Day 7 – Saturday

Breakfast: Vegetable and Turmeric Muffins

With a little more time on a Saturday, these eggy muffins hit the spot. They're endlessly adaptable to whatever vegetables you have lying around. They make a great family breakfast or brunch, and they freeze well if you have leftovers, so you can grab a couple for a weekday breakfast.

Serves 4

1 tbsp olive oil, plus extra for greasing

1 garlic clove, finely chopped

650g vegetables, finely chopped, sliced or grated (such as finely chopped pepper, grated carrot and courgette, sliced mushrooms and spinach)

8 eggs

2 tbsp chopped herbs (such as basil, tarragon, parsley and chives)

2 tsp turmeric

50g grated Parmesan

butter or olive oil, for greasing

salt and ground black pepper

1 Preheat the oven to 190°C/375°F/Gas 5. Grease a muffin pan – I usually get 10 muffins out of this mixture, but it slightly depends on the mix of vegetables I use.

2 Heat the oil in a large frying pan over a medium heat and cook the garlic for 30 seconds, then add all the vegetables. Cook gently for 10 minutes until they've wilted and released lots of liquid. Leave to cool.

3 Beat the eggs in a large bowl, then stir in the herbs, turmeric and all but a couple of teaspoons of the Parmesan. Squeeze the liquid from the veg mixture and add the veg to the bowl. Stir well, season and divide between the prepared muffin cases. Sprinkle over the last of the Parmesan. Bake for 15 minutes or until golden brown and set.

Lunch: Roast Squash and Pepper Soup with Ras-el-Hanout and Halloumi Croutons

We all need a good soup in our repertoire and this is mine. The squash and peppers can go in the oven while you're cooking the muffins – just don't forget about them. Once they're done, the rest comes together quickly.

Serves 4
1 butternut squash, halved top to bottom and seeds removed
3 green or red peppers, halved and deseeded
1 tbsp olive oil
1 onion, roughly chopped
2 garlic cloves, roughly chopped
1 tbsp ras-el-hanout spice mix
100g split red lentils
1 litre vegetable stock
squeeze of lemon juice
200g halloumi cheese, cut into cubes
4 tbsp pumpkin seeds, toasted
salt and ground black pepper
chopped fresh herbs, to garnish

1 Preheat the oven to 190°C/375°F/Gas 5. Put the squash, cut-side down, in a roasting tin and roast for 40 minutes. Add the

peppers to the tray and roast for another 20 minutes, until the squash is completely soft and the peppers have collapsed. Leave to cool.

2 Heat the oil in a large saucepan over a medium heat and cook the onion and garlic for 5 minutes or until translucent. Add the ras-el-hanout, cook for 30 seconds, then add the lentils and stock.

3 Scrape the cooked flesh out of the butternut squash, rub the skin off the peppers, and add the squash and pepper flesh to the soup. Simmer for 20 minutes until the lentils are cooked. Blend in a blender or food processor until smooth.

4 Gently reheat the soup and add the lemon juice, and salt and pepper to taste. Meanwhile, fry the halloumi in a dry frying pan until crusted and golden. Remove from the pan and add the pumpkin seeds to the pan. Dry-fry over a medium heat for 3 minutes or until golden, tossing frequently. Be careful that they don't burn. Set aside. Ladle out the soup and top with the halloumi croutons, the pumpkin seeds and herbs.

Dinner: Spiced Salmon with Pomegranate Molasses

Salmon is a treat, especially if you can get wild salmon, so I've saved it for Saturday night. Adding a sweet–tart marinade makes it extra special. Wild salmon goes from underdone to overdone in what seems like seconds, so keep a careful eye on it.

Serves 4
4 salmon fillets, wild if possible
2 tbsp pomegranate molasses
2 tbsp orange juice
1 tsp sweet smoked paprika

1 tsp ground cumin

1 tsp ground sumac (optional)

1 tsp ground cinnamon

1 tsp ground coriander

2 tbsp olive oil

1 tsp salt

200g quinoa or freekeh

2 tbsp fresh pomegranate seeds

2 tbsp each chopped fresh coriander and mint

salt and ground black pepper

green leafy vegetable or salad, to serve

1 Preheat the oven to 180°C/350°F/Gas 4. Put the salmon in a roasting tin. In a bowl, mix together the molasses, orange juice, spices and oil. Season well with salt and pepper, and spread half the mixture over the salmon. Bake for 10–12 minutes until the salmon is opaque – but don't let it dry out.

2 Cook the quinoa or freekeh in a pan with three times the volume of water for 15 minutes or until tender, or according to the packet instructions. Drain in a sieve and stir through the remaining sauce and herbs. Serve with the salmon and a green vegetable or salad.

Sweet things

Age-well Chocolate Bark

Dark chocolate is an age-well superfood, packed with anti-oxidants. This chocolate bark packs in more healthy ingredients and looks very pretty.

Makes about 4 portions
100g 70% dark chocolate, broken into squares
1 tsp coconut oil
1 tsp maple syrup
3 tbsp dried cherries or cranberries, or both
1 tbsp bee pollen
3 tbsp chopped nuts, Brazil nuts are a favourite of mine

1 Line a baking sheet with baking parchment. Melt the chocolate, coconut oil and maple syrup in a heatproof bowl over a
   pan of gently simmering water, making sure the base of the
   bowl doesn't touch the water.
2 Spread the melted chocolate mixture over the baking parchment and sprinkle with the dried fruit, bee pollen and chopped
   nuts. Allow it to cool before snapping into shards.

Peanut Butter and Dark Chocolate Squares

This is one of the most popular recipes on our blog, so I didn't
want you to miss out on it.

Makes 24 small squares
180g rolled oats
250g peanut butter
12 medjool dates, pitted
60ml maple syrup
2 tbsp coconut oil, melted
½ tsp vanilla extract
a good pinch of sea salt – don't skimp on this, it really brings
   the flavours together
150g 70% dark chocolate, broken into squares

1 Line a brownie pan with baking parchment. Blitz all the ingredients, except the chocolate, in a food processor until the mixture is sticky and clumps together when you pinch a small lump. Tip into a lined brownie pan and press down hard to smooth it out. Put in the freezer.

2 Melt the chocolate in a heatproof bowl over a pan of gently simmering water, making sure the base of the bowl doesn't touch the water. Pour the chocolate over the top of the peanut mixture and chill until needed. Cut into small squares (it's pretty rich) – and enjoy!

Banana, Oat and Choc-Chip Cookies

I buy bananas just so I can make these simple cookies. I've lost count of the number of times I've baked these over the years and I'm still thrilled to eat them every time.

Makes about 16 small cookies
3 ripe bananas
50g coconut oil, melted
125g oats
50g ground almonds
1 tsp vanilla extract
½ tsp salt
100g dark chocolate, chopped, or chocolate chips
50g dried cherries
50g walnuts, crumbled

1 Preheat oven to 170°C/350°F/Gas 4 and line two baking sheets with baking parchment. Mash the bananas in a large bowl and stir in the coconut oil. Stir in the remaining ingredients, making sure that they are all well distributed.

2 Dollop tablespoonfuls of the mixture onto the prepared baking sheets (these aren't going to be the most elegant biscuits you ever make). Bake for 15–18 minutes until the cookies are golden and any exposed bits of walnut look toasted.

Sauces

The vegetables, pulses and whole grains that form the backbone of age-well eating sometimes need a little pepping up with a well-flavoured sauce or dressing. Here are a few of my favourite 'flavour bombs'. They all take just seconds to make.

Punchy Herb Sauce

Makes 4 servings
4 tbsp olive oil
1 tsp finely chopped fresh rosemary
1 tsp finely chopped fresh thyme
2 tsp sweet smoked paprika
2 garlic cloves, finely chopped
2 tbsp tamarind paste
1 tbsp lemon juice
1 tsp dried chilli flakes
pinch of salt

Put all the ingredients in a small bowl. Stir well and season to taste with salt

Yogurt–Tahini Sauce

Makes 4 servings
4 tbsp natural live yogurt
2 tbsp tahini
juice of ½ lemon
1 garlic clove, finely chopped

Put all the ingredients in a bowl and beat well together, then add a little water to make a sauce that is slightly thicker than double cream.

Herb and Miso Green Goddess Dressing

Makes 4 servings
1 tbsp dark miso, or to taste
2 tbsp tahini
juice of 1 lemon, or to taste
1 tbsp maple syrup
3 tbsp roughly chopped fresh herbs (such as parsley, basil, coriander)
1 garlic clove, chopped

Put all the ingredients in a blender or food processor and add 3 tbsp water. Blend to make the sauce. Adjust the flavours to taste, adding more lemon or maple syrup if you need to.

APPENDIX IV

Household Cleaning Tips and Recipes

I've drastically reduced the number of harsh chemicals I use in my home, and instead use a small kit of 'ingredients' to mix up my own cleaning products. It's a fun and satisfying DIY project, and I say that as someone who used to *hate* cleaning. I've come to enjoy the process more because I'm in control of the products I use.

Do your homework before using any product, homemade or otherwise, on porous or specially treated surfaces.

Ingredients

Dr Bronner's Castile soap This all-natural liquid soap has been a revelation to me. It's super-concentrated, so one bottle lasts for ages, and it can be used for everything from cleaning the floor to cleaning your teeth. It's infused with a wide range of different essential oils, so choose one that appeals to you. I like tea tree for cleaning my home.

Bicarbonate of soda Baking soda and bicarbonate of soda are the same thing. Don't use the expensive little tubs from the baking section of the supermarket for cleaning: I buy 2kg bags of bicarbonate of soda on Amazon for around £7. Hardware stores also sell it.

Distilled white (household) vinegar This isn't a vinegar you'd cook with as it's way more acidic than, say, white wine, or balsamic, vinegar. But it's a powerful natural cleaning product and costs pennies. Don't use on marble or granite surfaces as it can damage the stone.

Essential oils I have a small armoury of essential oils – usually rosemary, tea tree and lavender – and add a couple of drops to my homemade cleaning products to make them smell wonderful.

Bottles and labels To make the all-purpose and glass cleaners you'll need spray bottles. They're readily available, and cheap, online or in kitchen shops. Don't forget to label any cleaning product you make with its ingredients and purpose.

Recipes

All-purpose Spray

> 2 tbsp Dr Bronner's Castile soap
> 500ml distilled or boiled water
> Few drops of essential oil
> Spray bottle and label

Mix the ingredients in the bottle and give it a good shake. Spray the surface you want to clean (I use this for my kitchen work-tops), wipe with a damp cloth, then finish with a dry one.

Glass Spray

> 250ml water
> 250ml white vinegar
> A few drops of essential oil
> Spray bottle and label

Mix the ingredients in the bottle and give it a good shake. Spray onto windows and other glass surfaces and polish dry with a soft cloth.

Oven Cleaner

> 120g bicarbonate of soda
> 3–4 tbsp water
> Glass spray (as above)

Remove all oven racks and grill pans from your oven and wash separately. Mix the bicarbonate of soda and water into a smooth paste. Using rubber gloves, smear the paste all over the inside of the oven (avoiding the heating elements), working it into any nooks and crannies. Leave overnight to work its magic. Use an old, damp dishcloth to wipe out the paste residue, scraping up any residue as you go. Spritz the glass spray onto any remaining paste (the acid will react with the bicarbonate to create foam, making it easier to remove) and give your oven a final wipe down.

Floor Cleaner

> 4 tbsp Dr Bronner's Castile soap
> Approx. 10 litres hot water (which is what my mop
>   bucket holds)

Pop the soap into your bucket, fill up with hot water, and mop away!

'Bleach'

> 65g bicarbonate of soda
> 1 tbsp Dr Bronner's Castile soap
> Drop of essential oil (optional)

Mix to a paste with a little water and scrub round loos, baths and sinks.

Dishwasher Cleaner

Once a month I run my dishwasher with a cup of distilled white vinegar on the top rack. This removes any gunky build-up and leaves the machine sparkling clean.

Also in my kit

Coconut scrubbies, loofah washing up pads, microfibre e-cloths, magic paint cleaners (not plastic free but they clean dirty marks off paintwork without chemicals).

Brands to Try

If making your own cleaning products is a step too far, there are lots of good 'clean' cleaning products on the market that will reduce the chemical load in your home:

Method: very widely available and a market leader since 2000. The anti-bacterial all-purpose cleaner does just about everything.

Ecover: also very widely available. I like the laundry products and washing up liquid.

Bio D: a large range of environmentally-friendly cleaning products. They're often sold in bulk so can be good value, and all are made in England. I particularly like the floor cleaner.

Tincture: expensive but so beautifully packaged and scented with essential oils that you'll feel like you're washing up in a spa. I have been known to give these cleaning products to girlfriends as gifts!

References

In the process of writing this book I consulted numerous sources of information (mostly academic research papers). These sources are acknowledged with a number in the relevant place in the text, so that you can delve deeper if you wish. In order to save paper (there are more than a hundred cited sources). I have placed the corresponding details of the citations on the Age Well Project website (agewellproject.com).

Further reading, podcasts and websites

Books

These are just some of the sources that have inspired me.

The Changing Mind by Daniel Levitin
Life Lessons from a Brain Surgeon by Rahul Jandial
Fiber Fueled by Dr Will Bulsiewicz
Why We Sleep by Matthew Walker
The Art of Sleeping by Rob Hobson
Chasing the Sun by Linda Geddes
Extra Time by Camilla Cavendish
Lifespan by David Sinclair
The Circadian Code by Satchin Panda
Food: WTF Should I Eat by Dr Mark Hyman
Growing Young by Marta Zaraska
Eat to Beat Disease by Dr William Li
Self-Care for the Soul by Jody Shield
Low Tox Life by Alexx Stuart
Growing Older Without Feeling Old by Rudi Westendorp
The Organised Mum Method by Gemma Bray
Feast on Phytochemicals by Paul Williams
The XX Brain by Lisa Mosconi

Podcasts

I'm always listening to podcasts, either when I'm getting my daylight on a walk or striding round the park with my dogs (black coffee in hand!).

Found my Fitness – Rhonda Patrick

Fad or Future – Joey Thurman

The Natural Healthcare Network – Deb MacLeod

She's Electric – Jody Shield

The BMJ

The Doctor's Kitchen – Dr Rupy Aujla

Ben Greenfield Fitness

Feel Better, Live More

The Plant Proof Podcast

The Rich Roll Podcast

Deliciously Ella

How to Fail – Elizabeth Day

Websites and Online Shops

Foundmyfitness.com

https://positiveageing.org.uk

www.positivepsychology.com

https://lifespanbook.com

www.medicalnewstoday.com

www.nhs.uk

www.pubmed.com

https://www.nature.com

Mindbodygreen.com

https://medium.com

https://www.who.int

http://apoe4.info

www.alittlefind.com – green beauty and home care products

www.lisabronner.com – granddaughter of the original Dr Bronner – somewhat biased towards the products, of course, but a great resource for natural bathing and home cleaning

www.ethicalsuperstore.com – good range of environmentally-friendly cleaning products

Index